THE EVIL EYE

THANATOLOGY AND OTHER ESSAYS

First Edition 1912
Roswell Park

New Edition 2019
Edited by Tarl Warwick

COPYRIGHT AND DISCLAIMER

FOREWORD

This following work is, in essence, one part occult and one part strictly scientific in nature, being predominantly a historical and medical work, those fields necessitating largely religious content. Indeed, even the mundane content here (such as in the section regarding the history of anesthesia, and the timeline there of the development of nitrous oxide, ether, and the like) intertwines at least at most times with organized religion, which the scientific minds of the day were growing more hostile towards and which here are criticized with fair regularity. It is possible to fine this collection of essays and speeches somewhat amusing for some of its content- both the sarcastic remarks on the Catholic church, as well as its advocacy for the use of cocaine in the field of pain relief- which almost renders dating the work unnecessary since it was only in vogue for a few decades around this particular period in the early 20th century.

The first two essays here are of the greatest importance perhaps for strictly occult importance beyond the topical need for those practicing the same to acknowledge and understand history (and often medicine, at least with regards to herbal healing and similar facets of many spiritual systems.) The concept of the evil eye- of fixation and of mesmerism after a fashion, and its importance especially within Italian and Italy-derived traditions is both interesting and highly relevant- the basic concept remains in use today, and has long since seeped out from Italy (and Italian communities in the new world) into regular use- the Charles Leland-esque section thereupon here is dense but good.

Thanatology, the second section, is also of great interest and delves in the most essential sense into the philosophical and biological argument that continues even now over what specifically constitutes the nature of life (in multiple senses.) A person thus is said to be alive, but should even a fairly large proportion of their biological tissue become rotten and die, it is possible for the human, as a whole, to remain alive- does only cognition itself matter and, if so, how are non-cognitive life forms to be considered life at all? The bio-ethical dilemma is explored in depth there.

The work continues, relating as well the intriguing history of surgery as a profession and its technical origins in the European sense with barbers- indeed, those who shave beards and heads of hair, and with a long treatment of the history of the Knights Hospitaller and their latter day descendants (which indeed still operate.)

This edition of "The Evil Eye, Thanatology, and Other Essays" has been carefully edited for format and content. Care has been taken to retain all original intent and meaning.

THE EVIL EYE, THANATOLOGY, AND OTHER ESSAYS

PREFACE

Responsibility for the following collection of essays and addresses (occasional papers) rests perhaps not more with their writer, who was not unwilling to see them presented in a single volume, than with those of his friends who were complimentary enough to urge their assemblage and publication in this shape.

They partake of the character of studies in that border-land of anthropology, biology, philology and history which surrounds the immediate domain of medical and general science. This ever offers a standing invitation and an enduring fascination for those who will but raise their eyes from the fertile and arable soil in which they concentrate their most arduous labors. Too close confinement in this field may result in greater commercial yield, but the fragrance of the clover detracts not at all from the value of the hay, nor do borderland studies result otherwise than in enlargement of the boundaries of one's storm center of work. No strictly technical nor professional papers have been reprinted herein, while several of those which appear do so for the first time.

Buffalo, December, 1912.

THE EVIL EYE

I: THE EVIL EYE

Belief in magic has been called by Tylor, one of the greatest authorities on the occult sciences, "one of the most pernicious delusions that ever vexed mankind." It has been at all times among credulous and superstitious people made the tool of envy, which Bacon well described as the vilest and most depraved of all feelings. Bacon, moreover, singled out love and envy as the only two affections which have been noted to fascinate, or bewitch, since they both have "vehement wishes, frame themselves readily into imaginations and suggestions and come easily into the eye." He also noted the fact that in the Scriptures envy was called the Evil Eye.

It is to this interesting subject in anthropological and folk-lore study, namely, the Evil Eye, that I wish to invite your attention for a time. Belief in it is, of course, inseparable from credence in a personal devil or some personal evil and malign influence, but in modern times and among people who are supposed to be civilized has been regarded ordinarily as an attribute of the devil. Consideration of the subject is inseparable, too, from a study of the expressions "to fascinate" and "to bewitch." Indeed this word "fascination" has a peculiar etymological interest. It seems to be a Latin form of the older Greek verb "baskanein" or else to be descended from a common root. No matter what its modern signification, originally it meant to bewitch or to subject to an evil influence, particularly by means of eyes or tongue or by casting of spells. Later it came to mean the influencing of the imagination, reason or will in an uncontrollable manner, and now, as generally used, means to captivate or to allure. Its use in our language is of itself an indication of the superstition so generally prevalent centuries ago. It is, however, rather a polite term for which we have the more vulgar equivalent "to bewitch," used in a signification much more like the original meaning.

THE EVIL EYE

Belief in an evil power constantly at work has existed from absolutely prehistoric times. It has been more or less tacitly adopted and sanctioned by various creeds or religious beliefs, particularly so by the church of Rome, by medieval writers and by writers on occult science. Even now it exists not only among savage nations but everywhere among common people. We today may call it superstition, but there was a time when it held enormous sway over mankind, and exercised a tremendous influence. In its present form it consists often of a belief that certain individuals possess a blighting power, and the expression in England to "overlook" is not only very common, but an easily recognizable persistence of the old notion. Evidently St. Paul shared this prevalent belief when he rebuked the foolish Galatians, saying as in our common translation, "Who hath bewitched you that ye should not obey the truth?" In the Vulgate the word translated "bewitch" is "fascinare," exactly the same word as used by Virgil, and referring to the influence of the evil eye. Cicero himself discussed the word "fascination," and he explained the Latin verb *invidere* and noun *invidia* as meaning to look closely at; whence comes our word envy, or evil eye.

All the ancients believed that from the eyes of envious or angry people there was projected some malign influence which could infect the air and penetrate and corrupt both living creatures and inanimate objects. Woyciki, in his Polish Folk-lore, relates the story of a most unhappy Slav, who though possessed of a most loving heart realized that he was afflicted with the evil eye, and at last blinded himself in order that he might not cast a spell over his children. Even today, among the Scotch Highlanders, if a stranger look too admiringly at a cow the people believe that she will waste away of the evil eye, and they give him of her milk to drink in order to break the spell. Plutarch was sure that certain men's eyes were destructive to infants and young animals, and he believed that the Thebans could thus destroy not only the young but strong men. The classical writers are so full of allusions to this subject that it is easy to see where people during the Middle Ages got their prevalent belief in witches. Thus, Pliny said that those possessed of the evil eye would not sink in water, even if weighed down with clothes; hence the medieval ordeal by water- which had, however, its inconveniences for the innocent, for if the reputed witch sank he evidently was not guilty, but if he floated he was counted guilty and then burned. Not only was this effect supposed to be produced by the fascinating eye, but even by the voice, which, some asserted, could blast trees, kill children and destroy animals. In Pliny's time special laws were enacted against injury to crops by incantation or fascination; but the Romans went even farther than this, and believed that their gods were envious of each other and cast their evil eyes upon the less powerful of their own circle; hence the caduceus which Mercury always carried as a protection.

To be the reputed possessor of an evil eye was an exceeding great misfortune. Solomon lent himself to the belief when he enjoined, "Eat thou not the bread of him that hath an evil eye." (Prov. 23:6). The most inconvenient country in which to have this reputation today is Italy, and especially in Naples. The Italians apply the term jettatore to the individual thus suspected, and to raise the cry of "Jettatore" in a Neapolitan crowd even today is to cause a speedy stampede. For the Italians the worst of all is the "jettatore di bambini," or the fascinator of infants. Elworthy relates the case of a gentleman who on three occasions acted in Naples in the capacity of sponsor; singularly all three children died, whereupon he at once got the reputation of having the "malocchio" to such an extent that mothers would take all sorts of precautions to keep their children out of his sight. The great Bacon lent himself also to the belief to such an extent as to advise the carrying on one's person of certain articles, such as rue, or a wolf's tail or even an onion, by which the evil influence was supposed to be averted.

A most interesting work was written by Valletta and published in Naples in 1787. It was practically treatise upon fascination and the jettatore. Valletta himself was a profound believer in all this sort of thing, and finished up his work by offering rewards for answers to certain questions, among which were the following: "Which jettatore is most powerful, he who has or he who has not a wig? Whether monks are more powerful than others? To what distance does the influence of the jettatore extend, and whether it operates more to the side, front or back? What words in general ought one to repeat to escape the evil eye?"

In ancient times it was believed that women had greater power of fascination then men, a belief to which our sex still hold at the present day, although in modern times the evil eye proper is supposed to be possessed by men rather than by women, monks especially, ever since the establishment of religious orders, being considered to possess this fatal influence. Curiously enough, the late Pope, Pius IX, was supposed to be a most pronounced jettatore, and the most devout Catholics would point two fingers at him even while receiving his blessing. Let me quote Elworthy in this connection: "Ask a Roman about the late Pope's evil eye, and he will answer, 'They say so, and it really seems to be true. If he had not the jettatura it is very odd that everything he blessed made fiasco. We did very well in the campaign against the Austrians in '48; we were winning battle after battle and all was gaiety and hope, when suddenly he blessed the cause and everything went to the bad at once. Nothing succeeds with anybody or anything when he wishes well to them. When he went to S. Agnese to hold a great festival down went the floor and the people were all smashed together. Then he visited the Column to the Madonna in the Piazza di Spagna and blessed it and the workmen. Of course one fell from the scaffold the same day and killed himself. He arranged to meet the King of Naples at Porto d'Anzio, when up came a violent gale and storm that lasted a week. Another arrangement was made and then came the fracas about the ex-Queen of Spain.'"

The superstition of the evil eye and of witchcraft goes

everywhere with the belief in the power of transformation, which at certain periods of history has been so prevalent as to account for many of the stories of ancient mythology, and will account even for such nursery stories as that of Little Red Riding Hood, as well as for the old-world belief in the werewolf.

Indeed, a common expression of today reminds one of this old belief, since it is a common saying to be ready to "jump out of one's skin for joy." This belief in transformation has begotten an ever-present dread of ill omens which is even now one of the most prevalent of superstitions. In Somerset, to see a hare cross the path in front of one is a sign of death. In India they fear to name any sacred or dreaded animal. The black cat is everywhere an object of aversion, and in some parts of England to meet a person who squints is equal to meeting one possessing the evil eye. Surely I do not need to remind this audience of the fear which many people have of taking any important action on Friday. This fear goes so far In some instances as to lead people to deprecate over-praise or apologize for a too positive statement. Your courteous Turk will not take a compliment without "Mashallah;" the Italians will not receive one without "Grazio a Dio;" while the Irishman almost always says "Glory be to God," and the English peasant "Lord be wi' us;" the Idea In every instance being to avert the danger of fascination by these acknowledgments of a higher power. In England during the horrible times when the Black Death raged It was supposed that the disease was communicated by a glance from the distorted eyes of a sick man. In 1603 Delrio, a Jesuit, published a large six-volume folio work entitled "A Disquisition on Magic," In which he takes It for granted that the calamities of mortals are the work of evil spirits. He says, "Fascination is a power derived by contact with the devil, who, when the so-called fascinator looks at another with evil intent, or praises by means known to himself, infects with evil the person at whom he looks." Those familiar with the history of so-called animal magnetism, mesmerism or hypnotism, will see a close connection between these beliefs and the practice of this peculiar form of influence.

THE EVIL EYE

Mesmerism, in fact, as ordinarily practiced, was more or less dependent upon the influence of touch, or actual contact, whose importance has always been by the credulous rated high. In fact, it will be remembered that many of the miracles of the New Testament were performed by the aid of touch, and in the Old Testament it is recorded how disappointed Naaman was when he went to be cured of his leprosy in that the prophet did not touch him. The influence of the royal touch for the cure of scrofula, known for centuries as the King's Evil, will also not be forgotten. In fact, our word to "bless" signifies to touch by making the sign of the cross on the diseased part, as, for instance, in the West of England, where goiter is rather common, it is believed that the best cure is that the swelling should be touched by the hand of a corpse of the opposite sex.

The more we deal with the superstitions now under consideration the more evident it becomes that the principal thought among the simpler peoples, or even among some of the religious sects of today, has been the propitiation of angry deities, or of destructive influences, rather than the worship and exaltation of beneficent attributes. As Elworthy says, "We find that fear and dread have in all human history been more potent factors In men's conduct than hope and gratitude or love." Take for example the propitiatory sacrifices of Abel and Cain, or the sacrifice which Abraham proposed to make of his own son, or the very words which have crept Into our language such as atonement, etc. With this personification of an evil power or attribute In nature came also belief in transformation, or metamorphosis, of which the Greek and Roman mythology Is full. How many of the Christian symbols of today, nearly all of which are of pagan origin, convey to the initiated Instances of this belief, can hardly be mentioned in this place. Suffice it to say that their number is very great. But I find too many temptations to wander from my subject, which is essentially the evil eye.

In medieval symbolism, as in ancient, the Intent often

was to represent either on some amulet, charm or picture a figure of the thing against which It was most desired that a protective Influence should be exercised, hence the general prevalence of the eye in some pictorial representation. The ancient Egyptians, as well as the Etruscans, used to paint a huge eye on the bows of their vessels, which was supposed to be a charm against the evil eye. Even today in the Orient I have seen Greek boats with eyes painted on either side of their prows. The eye was a common adornment of Egyptian pottery, usually in combination with various other pictures, but as a symbol it seems during the past century or two to have passed out of common employ, except perhaps in Malta, and among the Free-masons, who simply are perpetuating its use. Nevertheless, wax or silver eyes are seen hung up in some foreign churches. A curious feature of these superstitions has been this, that any feature of indecency or obscenity when attaching to these symbols, amulets, etc., has been supposed to make them much more potent. This probably was because anything strange or unusual was more likely to attract the eye, and therefore divert its influence from the individual to the inanimate object, hence the prevalence of phallic emblems in connection with these fancied protections. Many objects of this kind can be today picked up in the jewelry stores of Rome and of Naples.

Another of the most efficacious of these amulets takes the general form of a hideous mask, often called the Gorgoneion. In all probability this was largely for the reason given above- that it was most likely to attract attention. Symbols of this kind are In very general use among people who know nothing of the reason therefore. Thus, we see them on seals, coins, etc. The gargoyles of medieval architecture are frequently given this fantastic appearance and for this same purpose.

In Roman times the dolphin was a favorite device for a potent charm against the evil eye, and was pictured on many a soldier's shield. Ulysses adopted It as his especial choice, both on his signet and his shield, perhaps because it was supposed to have been through the agency of the dolphin that Telemachus was saved from drowning. To us in the medical profession it is of no little interest that in Rome, according to Varro, there stood three temples on the Esquiline dedicated to the goddess of Fever and one to Mephitis. Tacitus relates that a temple to Mephitis was the only building left standing after the destruction of Cremona, where there was also an altar dedicated to the Evil Eye. We know, also, that in the very center of the Forum there stood an altar to Cloacina, the Goddess of Typhoid. What complete sway this goddess has held from ancient times to the present I need scarcely tell you.

"When Rome, after the fall of the empire, relapsed into its most insanitary condition this old worship reappeared in another shape, and a chapel arose near the Vatican to the Madonna delta Fehre, the most popular in Rome in times of sickness or epidemic." This simply shows a transfer of ideas, the attributes of Diana being conveyed over to her Christian successor, the virgin, whose cult became equally supreme. The principal symbol of this cult was the horned moon or crescent, and, in consequence, horns in one form or another became the most common of objects as amulets against the Evil Eye. So comprehensive and persistent is this belief in Naples that, in the absence of a horn in some shape, the mere utterance of the name corno was supposed to be an effectual protection. Even more than this, the name Un Corno became applicable to any and every charm or amulet against the Evil Eye. We may find many references to the Horn in Scripture, where it served both as an emblem of dignity and as an amulet. Most curious it is that the phylactery with which the Pharisees adorned their garments, and which called forth the most scathing denunciation by the Master, was undoubtedly an emblem of a horn, and worn as an amulet against the Evil Eye. At the beginning of the Christian era it had become fashionable to wear these, and how they were enlarged and made not only badges of sanctity but marks of worldly honor, we may read in the New Testament.

THE EVIL EYE

The horn has been an important feature of Christian symbolism, as of pagan, and we constantly see the ram's horn, which was the successor of the bull's horn, made such from economical reasons, all over the ruins of ancient Rome. The married women of Lebanon wear silver horns upon their heads to distinguish them from the single women. The Jewesses of Northern Africa wear them as a part of their regular costume, and even today curious spiral ornaments are worn on either side of the head by the Dutch women. In Naples horns in all shapes are exceedingly common upon the trappings of the cab horses. Indeed the heavy trappings and harness of these overloaded animals are usually protected with a perfect battery of potent charms, so that any evil glance must be fully extinguished before it can light upon the animal itself. Thus, we may frequently see upon the backs of these animals two little brazen flags, said to be typical of the flaming sword which turned every way, and which are supposed to be an unfailing attraction to the eye. The high pommel ends usually in a piece of the inevitable wolf's skin, and many colored ribbons or worsteds are wound about portions of the harness in such a way as completely to protect all that it encloses.

But the most numerous of all these emblems is a hand in various positions or gestures. Probably every other cab horse in Naples carries the hand about him in some form. In Rome these things are not seen so much on horses' backs, although wolf skins, horns and crescents are common enough, but we see large numbers of silver rings for human fingers, to each of which a little pendant horn is attached. These may be seen in the shop windows strung upon rods and plainly marked Annelli contra la Jettatura. Those who have seen Naples thoroughly have noted how cows' horns, often painted blue, are fixed against the walls, especially at an angle, about the height of the first floor. But one of the most remarkable amulets which I have ever seen hangs outside one of the entries to the Cathedral in Seville, where over a door is hung by a chain the tusk of an elephant, and further out, over the same doorway, swung by another chain, an enormous crocodile, sent as a present or charm of special power to Alfonso, in 1260, by the Sultan of Egypt. These two strange charms hang over the doorway of a Christian church of today, indicating the acceptance by a Christian people of a Moslem emblem and amulet.

Again, in Rome it is very common to see a small cow's horn on the framework of the Roman wine carts or dangling beneath the axle. Much more common and better known among the Anglo-Saxon peoples is the horse-shoe emblem, which with us has lost all of its original signification, as an emblem of fecundity, and has become a charm against evil. It is hung up over doorways, is nailed up in houses, it guards stable doors and protects fields against malign influences. Even in the Paris Exhibition of 1889, where there was a representation of a street from old Cairo, there hung over several of the doors a crocodile with a horse-shoe on his snout. So far I have said very little about the positions of the hand and certain gestures by which it is intended to ward off the evil eye. The Mohammedans, like the Neapolitans, are profound believers in the efficacy of manual signs; thus outside of many a door in Tangier I have seen the imprint of a hand made by placing the outstretched hand upon some sticky black or colored material, which was then transferred as by a type or die to the doorway of the dwelling, where in the likeness of the outstretched manus it serves to guard the dwellers within. This is to me one of the most curious things to be observed in Mohammedan countries. A relic of the same belief I have seen also over the great gate of the Alhambra, in the Tower of Justice, where, in spite of the very strict Moslem custom and belief against representation of any living object, over the keystone of the outer Moorish arch is carved an outstretched upright hand, a powerful protection against evil. It is this position of the hand, by the way, which has been observed in all countries in the administration of the judicial oath. Moreover, the hand in this position is the modern heraldic sign of baronetcy.

THE EVIL EYE

The hand in the customary position of benediction is sometimes open and extended, while at other times only the first and second fingers are straightened. The power which the extended hand may exert is well illustrated in the biblical account (Exodus 17:11) "And it came to pass when Moses held up his hand that Israel prevailed, and when he let down his hand Amalek prevailed." And so it happened that when Moses wearied of the constrained position his hand was supported by Aaron and by Hur. This is only one of numerous illustrations in the holy writings showing the talismanic influence of the human hand. There are comparatively few people who realize, today, that the conventional attitude of prayer as of benediction, with hands held up, is the old charm as against the evil eye. In one of the great marble columns in the Mosque of St. Sophia in Constantinople there is a remarkable natural freak by which there seems to appear upon the dark marble the white figure of an outspread hand. This is held in the highest reverence by the superstitious populace, who all approach it to pray for protection from the evil eye. The open hand has also been stamped upon many a coin both in ancient and modern times, and the general prevalence of the hand as a form of doorknocker can be seen alike in the ruins of Pompeii and the modern dwelling.

The hand clenched in various forms has been used in more ways than as a mere signal or sign of defiance. In Italy the mano-fica implies contempt or insult rather than defiance. Among all the Latin races this peculiar gesture of the thumb between the first and second fingers has a significant name and a significant meaning. It is connected everywhere with the fig, and expresses in the most discourteous way that which is implied in our English phrase "don't care a fig." It is in common use as an amulet to be worn from the neck or about the body, and conveys the same meaning as that which the Neapolitans frequently express when they say "May the evil eye do you no harm." Another position of the hand, namely, that with the index and little fingers extended, while the middle and ring fingers are flexed and clasped by the thumb, gives also the rude imitation of the head of a horned animal, and is frequently spoken of as the mano cornuta. A Neapolitan's right hand is frequently, in some instances almost constantly, kept in that position pointing downwards, just as hand charms are made to hang downwards, save when It is desired to use the sign against some particular individual, when the hand is pointed toward him, even at his very eyes if he appear much to be dreaded. When, however, the hand in this position is pointed toward one's chin it conveys a most insulting meaning and hints at conjugal infidelity. As the Neapolitan cab-men pass each other the common sign is to wave the hand in gesture and in this position. This is true also of many other places.

The sign of the cross is very often made with the hand, usually with the first two fingers extended, and seems to mean a benediction of double potency, because both the hand and the cross itself are utilized in the gesture. I have elsewhere discussed the signification of the sign of the cross, and do not care to take it up again just now. It is certainly of phallic origin and as certainly antedates the Christian era by many hundred years. It is, in other words, a pagan symbol to which a newer significance has been given. Talismanic power has usually been ascribed to it, and in some form, either as the Greek Tau or the Crux Ansata, has been most frequently employed. In one or the other of these forms it was the mark set upon the houses of the Israelites to preserve them from the destroying angel. In the roll of the Roman soldiery, after a battle, it was placed after the names of those still alive; and we read in Ezekiel 9:4 of the mark which was to be set upon "the foreheads of the men that cry," which was certainly the Greek Tau, because the Vulgate plainly states this. Upon some of the old Anglo-Saxon coins there was placed a cross on each side, usually the handled cross, and upon various seals it has been in use until a comparatively recent period. It may be seen, also, in many illustrations from the catacombs, for instance, dating back to a time before the cross was a generally received Christian emblem, showing both the use of the cross and the hand in the positions to which I have already alluded.

THE EVIL EYE

The sign of the cross is made by many a schoolboy in his play before he shoots his marble, and I have often seen it made upon the wooden ball before a man has bowled with it. Many a peasant scratches it upon his field after sowing, and many a housewife has scratched it upon her dough. The hand with the first two fingers and thumb extended in the ordinary position of sacerdotal benediction was certainly a charm against evil long before the Christian era. This is not used so much by the common people, but has been appropriated rather by the priests. By a sort of general consent this has been especially the attitude permitted to the Second Person of the Trinity, although there are numerous instances in medieval painting where the hand of the First Person has been shown in this position. Indeed, the expression "dextera Dei" or "right hand of God," is conventionalized.

In many amulets, images and pictures, other charms are combined with that supposed to be exercised by the human hand. An exceedingly common one was the Egyptian scarab. The Egyptians believed that there were no females of this kind of insect, hence it was considered a symbol of virility and manly force, and in connection with the mano pantea just alluded to gave the amulet power to guard both the living and dead. In fact it was almost as common upon these emblems as the human eye itself. Again, the serpent was a frequent emblem in this same connection. As I have elsewhere written upon the subject of serpent-worship I need scarcely more than allude to it here, save to say that to the serpent were ascribed numerous virtues and powers, and that its use upon any charm was supposed to reinforce the virtues already possessed by it. Among the most curious of all the Italian charms against the Evil Eye, and yet one which has been singularly neglected by most writers, is the sprig of rue or, as the Neapolitans call it, the cimaruta. In its simplest form it was undoubtedly of Etruscan or Phoenician origin. Later, however, it became curiously involved with other symbols and quite complicated.

THE EVIL EYE

It is worn especially upon the breasts of Neapolitan babies, and is considered their especial protection against the much-dreaded jettatura. In ancient times no plant had so many virtues ascribed to it as had the rue. Pliny, indeed, cites It as being a remedy for 84 different diseases. It used to be hung about the neck in primeval times to serve as an amulet against fascination. In most of these amulet forms it consists of three branches, which were supposed to be typical of Diana Triformis, who used often to be represented in three positions and as if having three pairs of arms. Diana, by the way, was the especial protectress of women in child-birth. Silver was her own metal and the moon her special emblem. Therefore, the expression, "the silver moon" is not so meaningless as it would appear. This will in some measure account for the fact that corals, to which large virtues were ascribed, used always to be mounted in silver, and that the crescent, or new moon, is also almost invariably made of this same metal. Of the many charms which used to be combined in the cimaruta there is scarcely one which may not be more or less considered as connected with Diana, the Goddess of Infants.

Frequently, also, we may see representations of the sea-horse quite like the living hippocampi of today, which are worn alike by cab horses and by women in Naples. They are known locally as the Cavalli marini. Protection supposed to be most efficient was and is frequently afforded also by another method, namely, printed or written invocations, prayers, formulae, etc., worn somewhere about the body. Sometimes these were worn concealed from view and at others they were openly displayed. Even today on Turkish horses and Arab camels are hung little bags containing passages from the Koran, while the Neapolitan horses frequently carry in little canvas bags prayers to the Madonna or verses from scripture- these as a sort of last resort in case the other charms fail.

The good Catholic of today, especially if of Irish descent, wears his little scapulary suspended around the neck, which is supposed to be a potent protection. Frommannd's large work on Magic offers us a perfect mine of written spells against fascination, which have often to be prepared with certain mystic observances. The various written charms, as against the bite of the mad dog, are only other illustrations of the same superstition. Indeed, many superstitious people believe that the mere utterance of particular numbers exercises a charm. Daily expression of this belief we see in the credulity about the luck of odd numbers, and the old belief that the third time will be lucky. Military salutes are always in odd numbers. More value attaches in public estimation to the number seven than to any other, as we see in the miraculous powers ascribed to the seventh son of a seventh son. An appeal to luck today is the equivalent of the old prayer to the Goddess Fortuna, and is voiced in the common idea about the lucky coin and the various little observances for luck which are so popular. These observances are everywhere inclusive of the popular importance attached to expectoration, which is one of the most curious features of these many widespread beliefs. The habit of spitting on a coin, for instance, is very common, just as the schoolboy spits on his agate when playing marbles or on his baseball, or the bowler upon his wooden ball before rolling it. In fact, this whole matter of spitting has been in all ages an expression of a deep-rooted popular belief. Among the ancient Greeks and Romans the most common remedy against an envious look was spitting, hence it was called "despuere malum." Old women would avert the evil eye from their children by spitting three times (observe the odd number) into their bosoms.

The virtues and properties attributed to saliva among various peoples have been numerous and exalted. To lick a wart on rising In the morning used to be one of its well-recognized cures, and is today a popular remedy for any slight wound. Especially was the saliva of a fasting person peculiarly efficacious. Pliny states that when a person looks upon an infant asleep the nurse should spit three times upon the ground. But the most marvelous virtues were attributed to saliva in the direction of restoration of sight. The most conspicuous illustration of this is the instance mentioned in the New Testament when Christ healed the blind man, for it is related that: "He spat on the ground and made clay of the spittle, and did anoint the eyes of the blind man with the clay." The practice of concealing the eyes is prevalent throughout the Orient, and among the Mohammedans, cannot be referred entirely to male jealousy, for the women themselves confess to the greatest reluctance to show their faces to the stranger, fearing the Influence of the evil eye. Again, inasmuch as from time Immemorial diseases of all kinds have been considered the direct result of fascination, it was most natural that charms of varied form should be introduced as a protection. Many persons even of considerable education lend themselves to this superstition. The carrying in one's pocket of a potato, a lump of camphor or an amulet is, among other alleged charms, but an everyday illustration of this belief.

It would be possible to go on with an almost endless enumeration of the forms of this still generally prevalent belief in the power of the evil eye, and of the charms by which it may be averted. As has been set forth, it is but a particulate expression of a general and widespread belief in the existence of an evil being, for some vague and almost unsubstantial, for others assuming almost the proportions of the personal devil of medieval theology, or even of the Tyrolean Passion Plays. A discussion in a general way of this topic I have held to be not entirely foreign to the purpose of this society, it being one of the most interesting subjects of folklore study, and it may perhaps be considered just at the present to have a more particular interest for us in that we have so recently been favored with a most delightful and scholarly essay on the "Salem Witchcraft" by Prof. John Fiske, in which he graphically set forth the mechanism and the consequences of an aggravated expression of this belief, which constitutes the most serious blot which can be found upon the history of the Protestant white races in this country.

II: THANATOLOGY

A QUESTIONNAIRE AND A PLEA FOR A NEGLECTED STUDY

Appeared first in the Journal of the American Medical Association, April 27, 1912.

Is it possible to watch the "Vital spark of heavenly flame," as it quits "this mortal frame" and not be overcome by the mystery of death as the termination of that even greater mystery, life? Is there inspiration in the pagan emperor's address to his soul- those Latin verses which Pope has so beautifully translated?

To the speculative philosopher death may have a different significance, and one not altogether included in that given to it by the physiologist. To the former it is a subject for transcendental speculation; to the latter it is the terminal stage of that adjustment of Internal and external relations which, for Spencer, constitutes life. For us its primary and immediate significance is purely mundane, yet it deserves such serious study from a practical viewpoint as it seldom receives. What is death? When does it actually occur? How can it occur when the majority of cells in the previously living organism live on for hours or for days or, under certain favoring circumstances, retain potentialities of life for Indefinite periods? These and numberless related questions constitute a line of inquiry that may well call for a separate department of science. Pondering in this wise, I long ago coined an expression which years later I found had been Incorporated in the scientific dictionaries, though never before heard by me or encountered in my reading.

"Thanatology" is this word, and it may be defined as the study of the nature and causes of death. Inseparable from it, however, are certain considerations regarding the nature and causes of life. Yet I would not Introduce a compound term such as "biothanatology," wishing so far as possible to limit the study and the meaning. Let us ask ourselves a few more questions. Does life Inhere In any particular cell? In the leukocytes? In the neurons? Both are capable of stimulated activity long after the death of their host. In fact, by suitable electric stimulation, nearly all the phenomena of life may be reproduced after death, save consciousness and mentality alone. Do these then constitute life, and their suppression or abolition death? If so what about the condition of trance, or of absolute imbecility, congenital or induced? Or, again, how can a decapitated frog go on living for hours? Is it perhaps because the heart Is the vital organ that the hearts of some animals will continue to palpitate for hours after their removal from the bodies? Yet the animals which have lost them certainly promptly die. Suddenly stop a man's heart-action by electrocution, or the guillotine, or a bullet, and he dies, we say, instantly. Let it stop equally suddenly under chloroform and there is a period of several minutes during which it may be set going. Let a man apparently drown and this viable period becomes even longer- say a goodly fraction of an hour. During the interval is he alive or dead, or is there an intermediate period of absolutely suspended animation? And if so, in what does it consist? Is there a vital principle? If so what is it? Is such a thing conceivable? Can such a concept prevail among physicists? Can we consent even to entertain in this direction the notion of what is so vaguely called "the soul?" Of course, those who talk most lucidly about the soul know least about it, and no man can define it in comprehensible terms; but can consideration of the soul (whatever it may be) be omitted from our thanatology? Probably not, at least by many thinkers who cannot segregate their physics from their theology. Sad it is that theology, which might be so consolatory had it any fixed foundation, should be utterly impotent when so much is wanted of it. Theology, however, has little if aught to do with thanatology.

Is protoplasm alive? If so, then why may we not believe, with Binet, in the psychic life of micro-organisms? He seems to have advanced good reason for assuming that we may do so, albeit such manifestations in either direction may be scarcely more than expressions of chemotaxis. But if protoplasm be alive in any proper sense, as it would appear (else where draw the line?), just when does it so appear and whence comes its life? If it be alive, then life inheres in the nitrogen compounds composing it, or else is an adjunct of matter, imponderable, elusive, something conceivable if undeniable. The vitalists are of late perhaps attaining an ascendancy which for decades they had lost, since they maintain that life is not to be explained by chemical activities alone.

And yet it is possible to set going in the eggs of certain sea animals the phenomena of life, or to liberate them by certain weak solutions of alkaline cyanids, without the pressure or assistance of fructifying spermatozoa. In such cases life or death are determined by ionization and certain chemicals, or by their absence. Where then, again, is the vital principle? Or is it inherent in the ion, and was Bion correct when he said "electricity is life?" The life of a cell is then necessarily quite distinct from the life of its host, nor can the latter be composed simply of the numerical total lives of its components. Some lower animals bear semidivision, in which case each half soon becomes a complete unit by itself. Others seem to bear the loss of almost any individual part without loss of life, and it Is hard to say just which is the vital part. The central pumping organ is perhaps the sine qua non, when it exists. But when non-existent, then what? Again, while a living organism may be artificially divided Into viable portions, no method seems known by which a series of separate cells may be, as It were, assembled or combined Into one, of which a new unit may result from assemblage or combination. The more highly specialized or complex the cell, the more easily does it part with life, and the more difficult becomes Its preservation and Its reproduction. We may assume that after the death of a man his most specialized cells are the first to die, or more, that their death has perhaps preceded his own. In the ante-mortem collapse seen in many diseases and poisonings, has not this very thing occurred, i.e., that the patient has outlived his most important cells?

Certainly when a patient dies of progressive gangrene he has outlived, perhaps, a large proportion of his millions of competent cells. Viewed properly, what a strange spectacle is here presented! Perhaps twenty per cent, of his cells actually dead, the rest bathed In more or less poisonous media, still their host endures yet a little while. "Behold, I show you a great mystery." About which of the poisoned cells does the flame of life still flicker? The life-giving germ- and sperm-cells may exist and persist for some time after the body dies, as numerous experiences and experiments have shown. Ova and spermatozoa do not die the instant the host dies. And herein appears another great mystery, that cells from the undoubtedly dead body may possess and unfold the potentialities of life when properly environed. Among the lower forms of life cells but slightly differentiated go on living and even creating new organisms, though the larger organisms be dead. Moreover, in what way shall we regard the division of one ameboid cell into two, equally alive and complete? Here two living organisms are made out of one, without death intervening, and by permutation alone may one calculate, through how few generations cells need pass in order to be numbered by millions, without a death necessary to the process.

Thus far we have had in mind life and death in the animal kingdom alone. But most of what has been said, and much that has not, is equally true in the vegetable kingdom. Even in the mineral kingdom- as some think- the invariable and inevitable tendency to assume definite crystalline form represents the lowest type of life. Indeed it might fall in with Spencer's definition as evincing a tendency to adjust internal to external relations, though exhibited only after such ruthless disturbance as liquefaction by heat or solution. But then, is not every disturbance of relations "ruthless," because it follows inexorable habits of Nature? Even a crystal will reform as frequently as appear certain other phenomena of life, if made to do so. Were atoms alive they would suffer with every fresh chemical change, and who knows but that they do? But in the vegetable world we certainly have all the features of life and death in complete form: fructification of certain cells by certain others, development in unicellular form or in most profuse and complex form, a selection of necessary constituents of growth from apparently unpromising soil, and the production of startling results. Does not the sensitive plant evince a contact sensibility almost equal to that of the conjunctiva? And who shall say that it does not suffer when rudely handled? Does not the production of the complex essential oils and volatile ethers which give to certain flowers their wonderful fragrance, indicating what strange combinations of crude materials have been effected within their cells, show as wonderful a laboratory as any concealed within the animal organisms? Yet death comes to these plants with equal certainty, and presents equally perplexing mysteries. When dies the flower? When plucked and separated from its natural supply or when it begins to fade (a period made more or less variable by the care given it), or when it ceases to emit its odor? And is then death a matter of hours? When the floral stem was snapped what else snapped with it? At what instant did the floral murder occur?

Every seed and every seedling possesses marvelous potentiality of life, and so long as it does we say it is not dead; nor yet is it alive. It resists considerable degrees of heat, will bear the lowest temperature, will remain latent for long periods, and still its cells will instantly respond to favoring stimuli. Its actual life is apparently aroused by purely thermic and chemical (electronic?) activities environing it. In what do its life and its death consist? But life and death are influenced- we say "strangely" only because it all seems strange to us- by uncommon or purely artificial conditions. Radium emanations have always an injurious effect on embryonic development. Under their influence, for example, the eggs of amphibia become greatly disturbed. Cells that should specialize into nerve, ganglion and muscle fail to develop, and consequently there may be produced minute amphibian monsters, destitute of nerves and muscles, but otherwise nearly normal. Hertwig has submitted the sperm-cells of sea urchins to these rays, without killing them, but invariably with consequent abnormal development. The effect of cathode or X-rays is even more widely recognized and has been more generally demonstrated. They seem to possess properties injurious to most cell-life and even fatal to some.

Still more puzzling, and weird in a way, are the results of experiments, now widely practiced, which have to do with juggling, as it were, with ova, larvae and embryos, by all imaginable combinations of subdivision and reattachment of parts, so that there have resulted all kinds of monstrosities and abnormalities. To such an extent has this laboratory play been carried that almost any desired product can be furnished- living creatures with two heads, two tails, or whatever combination may be determined. Among the most remarkable of these efforts have been those of Vianney, of Lyons, who has shown that it is possible to remove the head end of several different insect larvae without preventing their development and metamorphosis into the butterfly stage. In *Bombyx* larvae, for example, the butterflies arrived at the mature stage, with streaked wings and beautiful coloration, but almost headless. These anencephalous insects lived for some time. Few animals survive exposures of any length to a temperature much over 150 F., and most of them are killed by considerably less heat. Freezing has always been considered equally fatal. Gangrene is the common result of freezing a part of the human body, and that means local death. Extraordinary pains must be taken with a frozen ear or finger if its vitality Is to be restored. And so even with the hibernating, or the cold-blooded animals, a really low temperature has been generally regarded as fatal.

But the recent experiments of Pictet, who did so much in the production of exceedingly low temperatures, freezing of gases, etc., have shown some startling results In the failure to kill goldfish and other of the lower animals by refrigeration. For instance, goldfish were placed in a tank whose water was gradually frozen while the fish were still moving therein. The result was a cake of Ice with imprisoned supposedly dead fish. This ice was then reduced to a still lower temperature, at which it was maintained for over two months. It was then very slowly thawed out, whereupon the fish came to life and moved In apparently their normal and natural ways as if nothing had happened. This confirms Pictet's early experiments and convictions, that if the chemical reactions of living organisms can be suspended without causing organic lesions the phenomena of life will temporarily disappear, to return when conditions are again as usual. It is worth relating that his fish frozen in this way could be broken in small pieces just as if they were part of the ice itself.

How often during these recent decades when events have seemed to move faster, when discoveries and inventions have been announced at such frequent and brief intervals that we fail to note them all for lack of time, when haste and rush characterize habits alike of life and thought, do we find that we simply must stop, as it were for breath, while we unload a large amount of accumulated mental rubbish and clear a space in our storage capacity for up-to-date knowledge! It is a decennial mental house-cleaning process. We must unlearn so much of that which ten to forty years ago we so laboriously learned. We must adopt new and improved reasoning processes. But it Is hard to do all this. For instance, as a boy I learned the old chemistry quite thoroughly. During a subsequent interval, when I did not need to study it, came the new chemistry, and when I again required it I had not only to study a practically new science- which was not so bad- but to rid my brain of much that had really found firm lodgment there, and this was difficult or impossible. So It is with one who, having been brought up on Euclidean geometry, finds himself confronted with the comparatively new non-Euclidean, and who has then not merely to forget, but to unlearn all those fundamental axioms which seemed so plain and so Indisputable, that is, if he would accept the teachings of Bolyai and others. For example, that a straight line Is not necessarily the shortest route between two points shocks our Euclidean orthodoxy, and is at the same time, to us, inconceivable; as also that parallel lines indefinitely prolonged may touch, and the like; likewise the concept of four-dimensional spaces, or worse yet, n-dimensional. And now, in somewhat like manner and to a certain degree, must we revise our previous conceptions of death, at least to this extent: Not that we yet know much better than we did what it really is, but that we know more about what it is not. Even save, perhaps, in its instantaneous happening it is hut a step toward dissolution, usually not the first, certainly not the last, but yet the most conspicuous.

Death is in many respects a biochemical fact. It is so intertwined with ionic changes in the arrangement of matter that we may hope for more Information regarding some of its aspects as knowledge of the latter accumulates. But, evidently, we need to clarify our notions as we rearrange our facts. Somatic death is, after all, a most complex process. It may be shortened by instant and complete incineration, but scarcely in any other way. Even dynamite would scarcely simplify the problem. As to conscious death, that is probably (though not certainly) a matter of seconds only or possibly fractions of a second. While we have no accurate appreciation of what constitutes consciousness, nor even just where it resides, the central nervous system appears to be its most probable seat. But conscious death may occur almost instantly without injury to this system, as when a bullet passes through the thorax and the heart, without injuring the spine.

But what is it that suddenly checks all concerted and interdependent activity? Or does something or some controlling agency suddenly leave the body? A recent theory, having features to commend it, is to the effect that life is a property or a feature of the ultimate corpuscles which compose the atom. Since these corpuscles bear to their containing atom a relative size comparable to that of the tiniest visible insect winging its way in a large church edifice, the intricacies of this particular theory readily appear. But it does seem as though among ourselves life has much to do with the hitherto neglected and despised nitrogen atom or molecule, since life inheres par excellence in nitrogen compounds. Moreover, vitality is conspicuously a feature of those chemical elements which have the lowest atomic weighty while at the other end of the table of atomic weights stands radium, of whose destructive emanations I have already spoken. Another phase of the general subject of thanatology was suggested especially by Osier, who a few years ago called attention to the fact that but few, if any patients really die of the disease from which they have been suffering. This is not a paradox, and needs only reason and observation to confirm it. His statement was a preliminary to the consideration of terminal infections and toxemias, which of itself would be sufficient to erect thanatology into a dignified special study. Take, for instance, a patient who has long suffered from diabetes. The end is characterized by coma, i. e., an evidence of profound toxemia, and is in large measure due to acetonemia. A patient with chronic Bright's disease dies of uremic poisoning, or one with pneumonia dies of genuine heart-failure. The terminal stage of cancer is, again, toxemia of one kind or another, according as it has interfered with digestion, with respiration, or some other vital function, or has broken down, thus saturating the patient with septic products.

This aspect of the subject will bear any amount of study and elaboration, and Its mention here should be sufficient for my purpose. Accordingly as it is properly appreciated, it will be recognized as having an important practical bearing, since, if we may foresee the direction from which the final danger threatens, it may be the better and the longer averted. Another very important and practical subject is wrapped up in this one, namely, the utilization of apparently dead, or at least of only potentially living material (tissue) in the various methods of grafting or transplantation, which are today a part of the surgeon's work. The methods are themselves a transplantation of experiences gained by work In the vegetable kingdom. What wonder that the marvels revealed in one department should have incited work along parallel lines in the other? That flowers and fruit of one kind may be made to grow on a tree of a very different kind excites but a small amount of the astonishment it deserves, mainly because it is now a common occurrence, though properly regarded it might seem a miracle.

Differing only in minor respect is, for example, the removal of thyroidal tissue from one human being and its implantation into another, with functional success. One may ask just here, how is this matter concerned with thanatology? And the reply is: If this tissue were taken from a fresh corpse it would be by most people regarded as dead tissue. If so, does the dead come to life? Without violating the proper scientific use of the imagination one may fancy something like the following: Let a healthy young woman meet accidental and instantaneous death. It would be possible to use no inconsiderable portion of her body for grafting or other justifiable surgical procedures. The arteries and nerves could be used, both in the fresh state, and the former even after preservation, for suitable transplantation or repair work on the vascular and nervous systems of a considerable number of other people. So also could the thyroid, the cornea, the ovaries and especially the bones. All the teeth, if healthy, could be reimplanted. With the thin bones, ribs especially, plastic operations- particularly on the noses- of fifty people could be made. And then the exterior of the body could be made to supply any amount of normal integument with which to do heterologous dermatoplastic operations, or would furnish an almost inexhaustible supply of epidermis for Thiersch grafts, which latter material need not be used in the fresh state, but could be preserved and made available some days and even weeks later. A portion of the muscles might possibly be made available for checking oozing from bleeding surfaces of others, if used while still fresh and warm, and possibly portions of the ureters or some other portion of the remains might be utilized for some unusual purpose. Then what extracts or extractives might be prepared from other parts of the body, pituitary, adrenals, bone-marrow, etc.? The tendons might also be prepared for sutures. Every one of these procedures would give promise of success, the technical being in every respect satisfactory.

But the possible limit is not yet reached, since with each kidney might be carried out experiments like those feats of physiologic jugglery such as Carrel has shown us, by implanting one, say in the neck, connecting up the renal with the carotid artery, and the renal vein with the jugular, while some receptacle would have to be provided as a terminal for the ureter. This is, after all, not a fantastic dream, nor such an extreme picture as would at first appear, since every organ or tissue above-mentioned- and more- has been used as indicated, and with success. But imagine the dead body affording viable products, even indirectly life itself, to (possibly) so many others! Does this complicate the study of death? And what must become of the simple credulous faith of the zealot who believes in the actual and absolute resurrection, at some later date?

There is something more than mere transcendental in the science of thanatology; it has a plausible edicolegal and pragmatic import. Right glad should I be if I might arouse a deserved interest in it. How may I more fittingly conclude than by quoting a few lines from our own Bryant's "Thanatopsis":

> "Earth that nourished thee, shall claim
> Thy growth, to be resolved to earth again,
> And, lost each human trace, surrendering up
> Thine individual being, shalt thou go
> To mix forever with the elements."

Though were I minded to rehearse certain difficulties met in the preparation of this paper, which I have long had in mind, I might also add the following lines from the same poet's "Hymn to Death":

THE EVIL EYE

"Alas ! I little thought that the stern power
Whose fateful praise I sung, would try me thus
Before the strain was ended."

One may well quote, at this point, Lamartine, who asked, "What Is life but a series of preludes to that mystery whose initial solemn note is tolled by death?" (On this theme Liszt built up that wonderful symphonic tone poem "Les Preludes.")

Even infinity is now questioned by the mathematicians. This being the case, where shall we, where can we stop?

Note: While writing the foregoing paper there came to my notice the recent book "Death; Its Causes and Phenomena," by Carrington and Header (London, 1911). It is interesting, but save that it contains a helpful bibliography, is of little assistance to one wishing to pursue the study from its pragmatic aspect. One of the authors is committed to a personal theory that death is caused by cessation of the vibrations which during life maintain vital activity; the other that death is, as it were, the culmination of a bad habit of expectancy that something of the kind must occur, into which we have fallen, in spite of the fact that other living beings below man undergo the same fate, though not capable of expecting anything.

THE EVIL EYE

III: SERPENT-MYTHS AND SERPENT WORSHIP

A Presidential Address before the Buffalo Society of Natural Sciences

Since the dawn of written history, and from the most remote periods, the serpent has been regarded with the highest veneration as the most mysterious of living creatures. Being alike an object of wonder, admiration and fear, it is not strange that it became early connected with numerous superstitions; and when we remember how imperfectly understood were its habits we shall not wonder at the extraordinary attributes with which it was invested, nor perhaps even why it obtained so general a worship. Thus centuries ago Horapollo referring to serpent symbolism, said: "When the Egyptians were representing a universe they delineated the spectacle as a variegated snake devouring its own tail, the scales intimating the stars in the universe, the animal being extremely heavy, as is the earth, and extremely slippery like the water; moreover it every year puts off its old age with its skin as, in the universe, the recurring year effects a corresponding change, and becomes renovated, while the making use of its own body for food implies that all things whatever which are generated by divine providence in the world undergo a corruption into them again."

In all probability the annual shedding of the skin and the supposed rejuvenation of the animal was that which first connected it with the idea of eternal succession of form, subsequent reproduction and dissolution. This doctrine is typified in the notion of the succession of ages which prevailed among the Greeks, and the similar notion met with among nearly all primitive peoples. The ancient mysteries, with few or perhaps no exceptions, were all Intended to illustrate the grand phenomena of nature. The mysteries of Osiris, Isis and Horus in Egypt; of Cybele in Phrygia, of Ceres and Proserpine at Eleusis, or Venus and Adonis in Phoenicia, of Bona Dea and of Priapus in

Rome, all had this sin common, that they both mystified and typified the creation of things and the perpetuation of life. In all of them the serpent was conspicuously Introduced as it symbolized and indicated the invigorating energy of nature. In the mysteries of Cercs, the grand secret which was communicated to the initiates was put In this enigma, "The bull has begotten a serpent and the serpent a bull," the bull being a prominent emblem of generative force. In ancient Egypt it was usually the bull's horns which served as a symbol for the entire animal.

When with the progress of centuries the bull became too expensive an animal to be commonly used for any purpose, the ram was substituted; hence the frequency of the ram's horns, as a symbol for Jove, seen so frequently, for example, among Roman antiquities. Originally fire was taken to be one of the emblems of the sun, and thus most naturally, inevitably and universally the sun came to symbolize the active, vivifying principle of nature. That the serpent should in time typify the same principle, while the egg symbolized the more passive or feminine element, is equally certain but less easy of explanation; indeed we are to regard the serpent as the symbol of the great hermaphrodite first principle of nature. "It entered into the mythology of every nation, consecrated almost every temple, symbolized almost every deity, was imagined in the heavens, stamped on the earth and ruled in the realms of eternal sorrow." For this animal was estimated to be the most spirited of all reptiles of fiery nature, inasmuch as it exhibits an incredible celerity, moving by its spirit without hands or feet or any of the external members by which other animals effect their motion, while in its progress it assumes a variety of forms, moving in a spiral course and darting forward with whatever degree of swiftness it pleases. The close relationship if not absolute identity among the early races of man between Solar, Phallic and Serpent worship was most striking; so marked indeed as to indicate that they are all forms of a single worship. It is with the latter that we must for a little while concern ourselves. How prominent a place serpent worship plays in our own Old Testament will be remarked as soon as one begins to reflect upon it. The part played by the serpent in the biblical myth concerning the origin of man is the first and most striking illustration. In the degenerated ancient mysteries of Bacchus some of the persons who took part in the ceremonies used to carry serpents in their hands and with horrid screams call "Eva, Eva;" the attendants were in fact often crowned with serpents while still making these frantic cries. In the Sabazian mysteries the snake was permitted to slip into the bosom of the person to be initiated and then to be removed from below the clothing. This ceremony was said to have originated among the Magi. It has been held that the invocation "Eva" related to the great mother of mankind; even so good an authority as Clemens of Alexandria held to this opinion, but Clemens also acknowledges that the name Eva, when properly aspirated is practically the same as Epha, or Opha, which the Greeks call Ophis, which is, in English, serpent. In most of the other mysteries serpent rites were introduced and many of the names were extremely suggestive.

The Abaddon mentioned in the book of Revelation is certainly some serpent deity, since the prefix Ab, signifies not only father, but serpent. By Zoroaster the expanse of the heavens and even nature itself was described under the symbol of the serpent. In ancient Persia temples were erected to the serpent tribe, and festivals consecrated to their honor, some relic of this being found in the word Basilicus, or royal serpent, which gives rise to the term Basilica applied to the Christian churches of the present era. The Ethiopians, even, of the present day derive their name from the Greek Aithiopes, meaning the serpent gods worshiped long before them; again, the Island of Euboea signifies the Serpent Island and properly spelled should be Oub-Aia. The Greeks claimed that Medusa's head was brought by Perseus, by which they mean the serpent deity, as the worship was introduced into Greece by a people called Peresians. The head of Medusa denoted divine wisdom, while the island was sacred to the serpent. The worship of the serpent being so old, many places as well as races received names indicating the prevalence of this general superstition; but this is no time to catalog names- though one perhaps should mention Ophis, Oboth, Eva in Macedonia, Dracontia, and last but not least, the name of Eve and the Garden of Eden.

Seth was, according to some, a semi-divine first ancestor of the Semites; Bunsen has shown that several of the antedeluvian descendants of Adam were among the Phoenician deities; thus Carthagenians had as God, Yubal or Jubal who would appear to have been the sun-god of Esculapius; or, spelled more correctly, Ju-Baal, that is Beauty of Baal. Whether or not the serpent symbol has a distinct phallic reference has been disputed, but the more the subject is broadly studied the more it would seem that such is the case. It must certainly appear that the older races had that form of belief with which the serpent was always more or less symbolically connected, that is, adoration of the male principle of generation, one of whose principal phases was undoubtedly ancestor worship, while somewhat later the race adored the female principle which they symbolized by the sacred tree so often alluded to in Scripture as the Assyrian grove. Whether snakes be represented singly, coupled in pairs as in the well known Caduceus or Rod of Esculaipius, or in the crown placed upon the head of many a god and goddess, or the many headed snake drinking from the jeweled cup, or a snake twisted around a tree with another approaching it, suggesting temptation and fall- in all these the underlying principle is always the same. Symbols of this character are met with not only in the temples of ancient Egypt but in ruins antedating them in Persia and the East; in the antiquities belonging to the races that first peopled what is now Greece and Italy, in the rock markings of India and of Central Europe, in the Cromlechs of Great Britain and Scandinavia, in the Great Serpent Mound which still remains in Ohio, and in many other mounds left by the mound builders of this country, in the ruins of Central America and Yucatan, and in the traditions and relics of the Aztecs and Toltecs- in fact wherever antiquarian research has penetrated or where monuments of ancient peoples remain. There never has been so widespread a superstition, and no matter what later forms it may have assumed we must admit that it, first of all, and for a long time was man's tribute to the great, all powerful and unknown regenerative principle of nature, which has been deified again and again, and which always has been and always will be the greatest mystery within the ken of mankind.

Brown in his "Great Dionysiak Myth" says the serpent has these points of connection with Dionysus, (1) as a symbol of and connected with wisdom, (2) as a solar emblem, (3) as a symbol of time and eternity, (4) as an emblem of the earth, life, (5) as connected with the fertilizing mystery, (6) as a phallic emblem. Referring to the last of these he says: "The serpent being connected with the sun, the earth, life and fertility, must needs be also a phallic emblem, and was appropriate to the cult of Dionysos Priapos." Again, Sir G. W. Cox says, "It is unnecessary to analyze theories which profess to see in it worship of the creeping brute or the wide-spreading tree; a religion based upon the worship of the venomous reptile must have been a religion of terror. In the earliest glimpses which we have the serpent is the symbol of life and of love, nor is the phallic cultus in any respect a cult of the full grown branching tree."

Again, "This religion, void of reason, condemned in the wisdom of Solomon, probably survived even Babylonian captivity; certainly it was adopted by the sects of Christians which were known as Ophites, Gnostics and Nicolaitans."

Another learned author says: "By comparing the varied legends of the East and West in conjunction we obtain a full outline of the mythology of the ancients. It recognizes as the primary element of things two independent principles of nature, the male and female, and these, in characteristic union as the soul and body, constitute the Great Hermaphrodite Deity, the one, the universe itself, consisting still of the two separate elements of its composition, modified though combined in one individual, of which all things are regarded but as parts." In fact the characteristics of all pagan deities, male or female, gradually mold into each other and at last into one or two; for as William Jones has stated, it seems a well-founded opinion that the entire list of gods and goddesses means only the powers of nature, principally those of the sun, expressed in a variety of ways with a multitude of fanciful names. The Creation is, in fact, human rather than a divine product in this sense, that it was suggested to the mind of man by the existence of things, while its method was, at least at first, suggested by the operation of nature; thus man saw the living bird emerge from the egg, after a certain period of incubation, a phenomenon equivalent to actual creation as apprehended by his simple mind. Incubation obviously then associated itself with creation, and this fact will explain the universality with which the egg was received as a symbol in the earlier systems of cosomogony. By a similar process creation came to be symbolized in the form of a phallus, and so Egyptians in their refinement of these ideas adopted as their symbol of the great first cause a Scarabaeus, indicating the great hermaphroditic unity, since they believed this insect to be both male and female. They beautifully typified a part of this idea also in the adoration which they paid to the water lily, or Lotus, so generally regarded as sacred throughout the East. It is the sublime and beautiful symbol which perpetually occurs in oriental mythology, and, as Maurice has stated, not without substantial reason, for it is its own beautiful progeny and contains a treasure of physical instruction. The lotus flower grows in the water among broad leaves, while in its center is formed a seed vessel shaped like a bell, punctured on the top with small cavities in which its seeds develop; the openings into the seed cells are too small to permit the seeds to escape when ripe, consequently they absorb moisture and develop within the same, shooting forth as new plants from the place where they originated; the bulb of the vessel serving as a matrix which shall nourish them until they are large enough to burst open and release themselves, after which they take root wherever deposited. "The plant, therefore, being itself productive of itself, vegetating from its own matrix, being fostered in the earth, was naturally adopted as a symbol of the productive power of the waters upon which the creative spirit of the Creator acted, in giving life and vegetation to matter. We accordingly find it employed in every part of the northern hemisphere where symbolical religion, improperly called idolatry, existed."

Further exemplification of the same underlying principle is seen in the fact that most all of the ancient deities were paired; thus we have heaven and earth, sun and moon, fire and earth, father and mother, etc. Faber says "The ancient pagans of almost every part of the globe were wont to symbolize the world by an egg, hence this symbol is introduced into the cosmogonies of nearly all nations, and there are few persons even among those who have made mythology their study to whom the mundane egg is not perfectly familiar; it is the emblem not only of earth and life but also of the universe in its largest extent."

In the Island of Cyprus is still to be seen a gigantic egg-shaped vase which is supposed to represent the mundane or Orphic egg. It is of stone, measuring thirty feet in circumference, and has upon it a sculptured bull, the emblem of productive energy. It is supposed to signify the constellation of Taurus, whose rising was connected with the return of the mystic re-invigorating principle. The work of the Mound Builders in this country is generally and widely known, still it is perhaps not so generally known how common upon this continent was the general use of the serpent symbol. Their remains are spread over the country from the sources of the Allegheny in N. Y. state westward to Iowa and Nebraska, to a considerable extent through the Mississippi Valley, and along the Susquehanna as far as the Valley of Wyoming in Pennsylvania. They are found even along the St. Lawrence River; they also line the shore of the Gulf from Florida to Texas. That they were erected for other than defensive purposes is most clear; without knowing exactly what was the government of their builders the presumption is that it combined both the priestly and civil functions, as obtained centuries ago in Mexico. The Great Serpent Mound, already alluded to, had a length of at least 1,000 feet; the outline was perfectly regular and the mouth was widely open as if in the act of swallowing or ejecting an oval figure, also formed of earth, whose longest diameter was one hundred and sixty feet. Again near Granville, Ohio, occurs the form of an alligator in connection with which was indubitable evidence of an altar. Near Tarlton, Ohio, is another earth work in the form of a cross. There is every reason to think that sacrifices were made upon the altars nearly always found in connection with these mounds. Among the various animal effigies found in Wisconsin, mounds in the form of a serpent are most frequently met with, while circles enclosing a pentagon, or a mound with eight radiating points, undoubtedly representing the sun, were also found.

There would seem in all these representations to be an unmistakable reference to that form of early cosmogony in which every vivification of the mundane egg constituted a real act of creation. In Japan this conceptive egg is allegorically represented by a nest egg shown floating upon an expanse of water, against which a bulb is striking with horns. The Sandwich Islanders have a tradition that a bird, which with them is an emblem of deity, laid an egg upon the waters, which burst of Itself and thus produced the Islands. In Egypt, Kneph was represented as a serpent emitting from his mouth an egg, from which proceeds the divinity Phtha. In the Bible there is frequent reference to seraphs; Se Ra Ph Is the singular of seraphim, meaning, splendor, fire or light. It is emblematic of the fiery sun, which under the name of the Serpent Dragon was destroyed by the reformer Hezekiah; or. it means, also, the serpent with wings and feet, as used to be represented in funeral rituals. Undoubtedly Abraham brought with him from Chaldea into lower Egypt symbols of simple phallic deities. The reference in the Bible to the Teraphim of Jacob's family reminds us that Terah was the name of Abraham's father, and that he was a maker of images. Undoubtedly the Teraphim were the same as the Seraphim; that Is, were serpent Images and were the household charms of the Semitic worshipers of the Sun-God, to whom the serpent was sacred.

In Numbers, 21, the serpent symbol of the Exodus is called a seraph; moreover when the people were bitten by a fiery serpent Moses prayed for them, when Jehovah replied, "Make them a fiery serpent, (literally seraph) and set it upon a pole, and it shall come to pass that every one who is bitten when he looketh upon it shall live." The exact significance of this healing figure of the serpent is far to seek. In this connection it must be remembered also, that among several of the Semitic tongues the same root signifies both serpent and phallus, which are both in effect solar emblems. Cronus of the ancient Orphic theogony, probably identical with Hercules, was represented under the mixed emblem of a lion and a serpent, or often as a serpent alone. He was originally considered Supreme, as is shown from his being called Il, which is the same as the Hebrew, El, which was, according to St. Jerome, one of the ten names of God. Damascius in his life of Isidorus mentions that Cronus was worshiped under the name of El. Brahm, Cronus and Kneph each represented the mystical union of the reciprocal or active and passive regenerative principles.

The Semitic Deity, Seth, was certainly a serpent god, and can be identified with Saturn and with deities of other people. The common name of God, Eloah, among the Hebrews and other Semites, goes back into the earliest times; indeed Bryant goes so far as to say that El was the original name of the Supreme deity among all the nations of the East. He was the same as Cronus, who again was the primeval Saturn. Thus Saturn and El were the same deity, and like Seth were symbolized by the serpent. On the western continent this great unity was equally recognized; in Mexico as Teotl, in Peru as Varicocha or the Soul of the Universe, in Central America and Yucatan as Stunah Ku, or God of Gods. The mundane egg was everywhere received as the symbol of the original, passive, unorganized formless nature, and later became associated with other symbols referring to the creative force or vitalizing influence, which was often represented in emblem by a bull. In the Aztec Pantheon all the other gods and goddesses were practically modified impersonations of these two principles. In the simpler mythology of Peru these principles took the form of the Sun, and the Moon his wife. Among the ruins of Uxmal are two long massive walls of stone thirty feet thick, whose inner sides are embellished with sculpture containing fragments of colossal entwined serpents which run the whole length of the walls; in the center of the wall was a great stone ring. Among the annals of the Mexicans the woman whose name old Spanish writers translated "The woman of our Fish" is always represented as accompanied by a great male serpent. This serpent is the Sun-God, the principal deity of the Mexican Pantheon, while the name which they give to the goddess mother of primitive man signifies "Woman of the Serpent."

Inseparably connected with the serpent as a phallic emblem are also the pyramids, and, as is well known, pyramids abound in Mexico and Central America. As Humboldt years ago observed pyramids existed through Mexico, in the forests of Papantha at a short distance above sea-level; on the plains of Cholula and of Teotihuacan, and at an elevation which exceeds those of the passes of the Alps. In most widely different nations, in climates most different, man seems to have adopted the same style of construction, the same ornaments, the same customs, and to have placed himself under the government of the same political institutions. Mayer describing one of his trips says, "I constantly saw serpents in the city of Mexico, carved in stone and in the various collections of antiquities."

The symbolic feathered serpent was by no means peculiar to Mexico and Yucatan. Squier encountered it in Nicaragua on the summits of volcanic ridges; even among our historic Indian tribes, for example among the Lenni Lenape, they called the rattlesnake "grandfather," and made offerings of tobacco to it. Furthermore in most of the Indian traditions of the Manitou the great serpent figures most conspicuously. It has been often remarked that every feature of the religion of the new world discovered by Cortez and Pizarro indicates a common origin for the superstitions of both continents, for we have the same worship of the sun, the same pyramidal monuments, and the same universal veneration of the serpent. Thus it will be seen that the serpent symbol had a wide acceptance upon this continent as well as the other, and among the uncivilized and semi-barbaric races; that it entered widely into all symbolic representation with an almost universal significance. Perhaps the latest evidences of the persistence of this belief may be seen in the tradition ascribing to St. Patrick, the credit of having driven all the serpents from Irish soil; or In the perpetuation of rites, festivals and representations whose obsolete origin is now forgotten.

For instance the annual! May-day festival, scarcely yet discontinued, is certainly of this origin, yet few if any of those who participate in it are aware that it is only the perpetuation of the vernal solar festival of Baal, and that the garlanded May-pole was anciently a phallic emblem. Among men of my own craft the traditions of Aesculapius are familiar. Aesculapius is, however, inseparably connected with the serpent myth and in statues and pictures he is almost always represented in connection with a serpent. Thus he is seen with the Caduceus or the winged wand entwined by two serpents, or, sometimes with serpents' bodies wound around his own; but rarely ever without some serpent emblem. Moreover the Caduceus is identical with the simple figure of the Cross by which its inventor, Thoth, is said to have symbolized the four elements proceeding from a common center. In connection with the Cross it is interesting also that in many places in the East serpent worship was not Immediately destroyed by the advent of Christianity. The Gnostics for example, among Christian sects, united it with the religion of the Cross, as might be shown by many quotations from religious writers. The serpent clinging to the Cross was used as a s3mibol of Christ, and a form of Christian serpent worship was for a long time in vogue among many beside the professed Ophites. In the celebration of the Bacchic mysteries the mystery of religion, as usual throughout the world, was concealed in a chest or box. The Israelites had their sacred Ark, and every nation has had some sacred receptacle for holy things and symbols. The worshipers of Bacchus carried in their consecrated baskets the mystery of their God, while after their banquet it was usual to pass around the cup which was called "The Cup of the Good Daemon," whose symbol was a serpent.

This was long before the institution of the rite of the Last Supper. The fable of the method by which the god Aesculapius was brought from Epidaurus to Rome, and the serpentine form in which he appeared before his arrival in Rome for the purpose of checking the terrible pestilence, are well known. The serpentine column which still stands in the old race course in Constantinople is certainly a relic of serpent worship, though this fact was not appreciated by Constantine when he set it up. The significance of the Ark is not to be overlooked. First, Noah was directed to take with him into the Ark animals of every kind. But this historical absurdity, read aright and In Its true phallic sense, means that the Ark was the sacred Argha of Hindu mythology, which like the moon In Zoroastrian teachings, carries in itself the germ of all things. Read in this sense the thing is no longer Incomprehensible. As En Arche (in the beginning) Elohim created the Heavens and the Earth, so in the Ark were the seeds of all things preserved that they might again repopulate the earth. Thus this Ark of Noah, or of Osiris, the primeval ship whose navigation has been ascribed to various mythological beings, was in fact the Moon or the Ship of the Sun, in which his seed is supposed to be hidden until it bursts forth in new life and power. But the dove which figures so conspicuously in the biblical legend was consecrated to Venus in all her different names, in Babylon, in Syria, in Palestine and in Greece; it even attended upon Janus in his Voyage of the Golden Fleece. And so the story of Jonah going to Joppa, a seaport where Dagon, the Fish-God was worshiped, and of the great fish, bears a suspicious relation to the same cult, for the fish was revered at Joppa as was the dove at Nineveh.

It has been impossible to dissociate serpent and serpent worship from Aesculapius. This is not because this mythological divinity is supposed to have been the founder of my profession, but because he has been given at all times a serpentine form and has been, apparently, on the most familiar terms with the animal. Pausanias, indeed, assures us that he often appeared in serpentine form, and the Roman citizens of two thousand years ago saw in this god "in reptilian form an object of high regard and worship." When this divinity was invited to make Rome his home, in accordance with the oracle, he is represented as saying:

> "I come to leave my shrine;
> This serpent view, that with ambitious play
> My staff encircles; mark him every way;
> His form though larger, nobler, I'll assume,
> And, changed as God's should be, bring aid to
> Rome."

(Ovid: Metamorphosis XV).

When In due time this salutary serpent arrived upon the island in the Tiber he began to assume his natural form, whatever that may have been; "And now no more the drooping city mourns, Joy is again restored and health returns."

Considering then the intimate relation between the founder of medicine and the serpent it will not seem strange to you that the serpent myth is a subject of keen interest to every student of the history of medicine. This devotion to serpent worship appears to have lingered a long time in Italy, for so late as the year 1001 a bronze serpent on the basilica of St. Ambrose was worshiped. De Gubernatis speaking of it says, "Some say it was the serpent Aesculapius, others Moses, others that it was the image of Christ; for us it is enough to remark that it was a mythological serpent before which the Milanese mothers offered their children when they suffered from worms, in order to relieve them," a practice which was finally suppressed by San Carlo. Moreover, there has persisted until recently what is called a snake festival in a little mountain church near Naples, where those participating carry snakes around their persons, the purpose of the festival being to preserve the participants from poison and sudden death and bring them good fortune. (Sozinskey).

The power of the sun over health and disease was long ago recognized in the old Chaldean hymn in which the sun is petitioned thus:

"Thou at thy coming cure the race of man;
Cause the ray of health to shine upon him;
Cure his disease."

Probably some feeling akin to that voiced In this way gave rise to the following beautiful passage in Malachi (4:2): "The Sun of Righteousness shall arise with healing in His wings."

As a purely medical symbol the serpent is meant to symbolize prudence; long ago men were enjoined to be "As wise as serpents" as well as harmless as doves. In India the serpent is still regarded as a symbol of every species of learning. It has also another medical meaning, namely, convalescence, for which there is afforded some ground in the remarkable change which it undergoes every spring from a state of lethargy to one of active life. According to Ferguson, the experience of Moses and the Children of Israel with brazen serpents led to the first recorded worship paid to the serpent, which is also noteworthy, since the cause of this adoration is said to have been its intrinsic healing power.

THE EVIL EYE

The prototype of the brazen serpent of Moses in latter times was the Good Genius, the Agathodaemon of the Greeks, which was regarded always with the greatest favor and usually accorded considerable power over disease. The superstitious tendency to regard disease and death as the visitation of a more or less capricious act by some extra mundane power persists even to the present day. For example, in the Episcopal book of Common Prayer, it is stated, in the Order for the Visitation of the Sick, "Wherefore, whatsoever your sickness be, know you certainly that it is God's visitation," while for relief the following sentiment is formulated in prayer, "Lord look down from heaven, behold, visit and relieve these, thy servants," thus voicing the very ideas which were current among various peoples of remote antiquity and eliminating all possibility of such a thing as the regulation of disease or of sanitary medicine.

IV: IATRO-THEURGIC SYMBOLISM

*An Address before the Maine Medical Association, Portland,
June 2nd, 1898*

So soon as had subsided the feeling of surprise, caused by a most unexpected invitation to address you tonight, I began at once to cast about for a subject with which I might endeavor so to interest you as to justify the high and appreciated compliment which this invitation mutely conveyed. And so, after considerable reflection, it appeared to me that it was perhaps just as well that medical men should be entertained, even at such a gathering as this, by something which if not of the profession was at least for the profession, and still not too remote from the purposes which have drawn us together. Accordingly I decided to forsake the beaten path and, instead of selecting a topic in pathology or in surgery, upon which I could possibly speak with some familiarity, to invite your attention to a subject which has always been of the greatest interest to me, yet upon which it has been hard, without great labor and numerous books, to get much information. If I were to attempt to formulate this topic under a distinctive name I could perhaps call it Medico-Christian Symbolism, It is well known to scholars that practically all of the symbols and symbolism of Christianity have come from pagan sources, having been carried over, as one might say, across the line of the Christian era, from one to the other, in the most natural and unavoidable way, although most of these symbols and caricatures have more or less lost their original signification and have been given another of purely Christian import.

To acknowledge that this is so is to cast no slur upon Christianity; it is simply recording an historical fact. It would take me too far from my purpose tonight were I to go into the reasons which brought about this change; I simply want to disavow all intention of making light of serious things, or of reflecting in any way upon the nobility of the Christian Church,

Its meanings or its present practices. But, accepting the historical fact that Christian symbols were originally pagan caricatures, I want to ask you to study with me for a little while the original signification of these pagan symbols, feeling that I can perhaps, interest you in such a study providing that it can be shown that almost all of these emblems had originally an essentially medical significance, referring in some way or other either to questions of health and disease, or else to the deeper question of the origin of mankind and the great generative powers of nature, at which physicians today wonder as much as they did two thousand years ago. Considering then the medical significance of such study I have been tempted to incur the charge of being pedantic and have coined the term Iatro-Theurgic Symbolism, which title I shall give to the essay which I shall present to you tonight.

As Inman says, "Moderns who have not been initiated in the sacred mysteries and only know the emblems considered sacred, have need of both anatomical knowledge and physiological lore ere they can see the meaning of many signs." The emblems or symbols then, to which I shall particularly allude, are the Cross, the Tree and Grove, the Fish, the Dove, and the Serpent. And first of all the Cross, about which very erroneous notions prevail. It is seen everywhere either as a matter of personal or church adornment, or as an architectural feature, and everywhere the impression prevails that it is exclusively a Christian symbol. This, however, is the grossest of errors, for the world abounds in cruciform symbols and monuments which existed long before Christianity was thought of. It is otherwise however with the Crucifix which is, of course, an absolutely Christian symbol. The image of a dead man stretched out upon the Cross is a purely Christian addition to a purely pagan emblem, though some of the old Hindu crosses remind one of it very powerfully. No matter upon which continent we look we see everywhere the same cruciform sign among peoples and races most distinct. There perhaps has never been so universal a symbol, with the exception of the serpent. Moreover the cross is a sort of international feature, and is spoken of in its modifications as St. Andrew's, St. George's, the Maltese, the Greek, the Latin, etc. Probably because of its extreme simplicity the ages have brought but little change in its shape, and the bauble of the jeweler of today is practically the same sign that the ancient Egyptian painted upon the mummy cloth of his sacred dead. Thus it will appear that the shadow of the Cross was cast far back into the night of ages. The Druids consecrated their sacred oak by cutting it into the shape of a cross, and when the natural shape of the tree was not sufficient it was pieced out as the case required. When the Spaniards invaded this continent they were overcome with surprise at finding the sign of the Cross everywhere in common use. It was by the community of this emblem between the two peoples that the Spaniards enjoyed a less war-like reception than would otherwise have been accorded to them.

That the Cross was originally a phallic emblem is proven, among other things, by the origin of the so-called Maltese Cross, which originally was carved out of solid granite, and represented by four huge phalli springing from a common center, which were afterward changed by the Knights of St. John of Malta into four triangles meeting at a central globe; thus we see combined the symbol of eternal and the emblem of constantly renovating life. The reason why the Maltese Cross had so distinctly a phallic origin, and why the Knights of St. John saw fit to make something more decent of it, is not clear, but a study of Assyrian antiquities of the days of Nineveh and Babylon shows that it referred to the four great gods of the Assyrian Pantheon, and that with a due setting it signifies the sun ruling both the earth and heavens. Schliemann discovered many examples of it on the vases which he exhumed from the ruins of Troy. But probably the most remarkable of all crosses is that which is exceedingly common upon Egyptian monuments and is known as the Crux-Ansata, that is the handled cross, which consisted of the ordinary Greek Tau or cross, with a ring on the top. When the Egyptian was asked what he meant by this sign he simply replied that it was a divine mystery, and such it has largely remained ever since. It was constantly seen in the hands of Isis and Osiris. In nearly the same shape the Spaniards found it when they first came to this continent. The natives said that It meant "Life to come."

In the British Museum one may see, In the Assyrian galleries, effigies In stone of certain kings from whose necks are suspended sculptured Maltese crosses, such as the Catholics call the Pectoral Cross. In Egypt, long before Christ, the sacred Ibis was represented with human hands and feet, holding the staff of Isis in one hand and the Cross in the other. The ancient Egyptian astronomical signs of planets contained numerous crosses. Saturn was represented by a cross surmounting a ram's horn; Jupiter by a cross beneath a horn, Venus by a cross beneath a circle (practically the Crux-Ansata), the Earth by a cross within the circle, and Mars by a circle beneath the cross; many of these signs are in use today. Between the Buddhist crosses of India and those of the Roman church are remarkable resemblances; the former were frequently placed upon a Calvary as is the Catholic custom today. The cross is found among the hieroglyphics of China and upon Chinese pagodas, and upon the lamps with which they illuminated their temples. Upon the ancient Phoenician medals were inscribed the Cross, the Rosary and the Lamb. In England there has been for a long time the custom of eating the so-called Hot-Cross Buns upon Good Friday- this is no more than a reproduction of a cake marked with a cross which used to be duly offered to the serpent and the bull in heathen temples, as also to human idols. It was made of flour and milk, or oil, and was often eaten with much ceremony by priests and people.

Perhaps the most ancient of all forms of the cross is the cruciform hammer known sometimes as Thor's Battle Ax. In this form it was venerated by the heroes of the North as a magical sign, which thwarted the power of death over those who bore it. Even today it is employed by the women of India and certain parts of Africa as indicating the possession of a taboo with which they protect their property. It has been stated that this was the mark which the prophet was commanded to impress upon the foreheads of the faithful in Judah. (Ezekiel 9:4).

It is of interest also as being almost the last of the purely pagan symbols to be religiously preserved in Europe long after the establishment of Christianity, since to the close of the Middle Ages the Cistercean monk wore it upon his stole. It may be seen upon the bells of many parish churches, where it was placed as a magical sign to subdue the vicious spirit of the tempest. The original cross, no matter what its form, had but one meaning; it represented creative power and eternity. In Egypt, Assyria and Britain, in India, China and Scandinavia, it was an emblem of life and immortality; upon this continent it was the sign of freedom from suffering, and everywhere it symbolized resurrection and life to come. Moreover from its common combination with the yoni or female emblem, we may conclude, with Inman, that the ancient Cross was an emblem of the belief in a male Creator and the method by which creation was initiated. Next to the Cross, the Tree of Life of the Egyptians furnishes perhaps the most ancient and universal symbol of immortality. The tree is probably the most generally received symbol of life, and has been regarded as the most appropriate.

The fig tree especially has had the highest place in this regard. From it gods and holy men ascended to heaven; before it thousands of barren women have worshiped and made offerings; under it pious hermits have become enlightened, and by rubbing together fragments of its wood, holy fire has been drawn from heaven. An anonymous Catholic writer has stated, "No religion is founded upon international depravity. Searching back for the origin of life, men stopped at the earliest point to which they could trace it and exalted the reproductive organs in the symbols of the Creator. The practice was at least calculated to procure respect for a side of nature liable, under an exclusively spiritual regime, to be relegated to undue contempt... Even Moses himself fell back upon it when, yielding to a pressing emergency, he gave his sanction to serpent worship by his elevation of the brazen serpent upon a pole or cross, for all portions of this structure constituted the most universally accepted symbol of sex in the world."

As perfectly consistent with the ancient doctrine that deity is both male and female take this thought from Proclus, who quotes the following among other Orphic verses: "Jupiter is a man; Jupiter is also an immortal maid;" while in the same commentary we read that "All things were contained in the womb of Jupiter." In this connection it was quite customary to depict Jupiter as a female, sometimes with three heads; often the figure was drawn with a serpent and was venerated under the symbol of fire. It was then called Mythra and was worshiped in secret caverns. The rites of this worship were quite well known to the Romans.

The hermaphrodite element of religion Is sex worship; gods are styled he-she; Syneslus gives an inscription on an Egyptian deity, "Thou art the father and thou art the mother; thou art the male and thou art the female." Baal was of uncertain sex and his votaries usually invoked him thus, "Hear us whether thou art god or goddess." Heathens seem to have made their gods hermaphrodites in order to express both the generative and prolific virtue of their deities. I have myself heard one of the finest living Hindu scholars, a convert to Christianity, invoke the God of the Christian Church both as father and as mother. The most significant and distinctive feature of nature worship certainly had to do with phallic emblems. This viewed in the light of ancient times simply represented allegorically that mysterious union of the male and female principle which seems necessary to the existence of animate beings. If, in the course of time, it sadly degenerated, we may lament the fact, while, nevertheless, not losing sight of the purity and exalted character of the original idea. Of its extensive prevalence there is ample evidence, since monuments indicating such worship are spread over both continents and have been recognized in Egypt, India,

THE EVIL EYE

Assyria, Western Europe, Mexico, Peru, Haiti and the Pacific Islands. Without doubt the generative act was originally considered as a solemn sacrament in honor of the Creator. As Knight has insisted, the indecent ideas later attached to it, paradoxical as it may seem, were the result of the more advanced civilization tending toward its decline, as we see in Rome and Pompeii. Voltaire speaking of phallic worship says "Our ideas of propriety lead us to suppose that a ceremony which appears to us so infamous could only be invented by licentiousness, but it is impossible to believe that depravity of manners would ever lead among any people to the establishment of religious ceremonies. It is probable, on the contrary, that this custom was first Introduced in times of simplicity, and that the first thought was to honor a deity in the symbol of life which it gives us."

The so-called Jewish rite of circumcision was practiced among Egyptians and Phoenicians long before the birth of Abraham. It had a marked religious significance, being a sign of the Covenant, and was a patriarchal observance because It was always performed by the head of the family. Indeed on the authority of the Veda, we learn that this was the case also even among the primitive Aryan people. Later In the centuries, as Patterson has observed, obscene methods became the principal feature of the popular superstition and were. In after times, even extended to and Intermingled with gloomy rites and bloody sacrifices. The mysteries of Ceres and Bacchus celebrated at Eleusis were probably the most celebrated of all the Grecian observances. The addition of Bacchus was comparatively a late one, and this name Bacchus was first spelled Iacchos; the first half, Iao, being in all probability related to Jao which appears In Jupiter or Jovispater, and to the Hebrew Yahve, or Jehovah. Jao was the Harvest God and consequently the god of the grape, hence his close relation to Bacchus. How completely these Elusinian mysteries degenerated Into Bacchic orgies is of course a matter of written history.

I have not yet alluded to the reverence paid to the fish,

both as phallic emblem and as a Christian symbol. The supposition that the reason why the fish played so large a part In early Christian symbolism was because of the fact that each letter of the Greek word Ichthus could be made the beginning of words which when fully spelled out, read Jesus Christ, the Son of God, etc.. Is altogether too far-fetched; though it be true it is a scholastic trick to juggle with words in this way rather than to find for them a proper signification.

Among the Egyptians and many other nations, the greatest reverence was paid to this animal. Among the natives the rivers which contained them were esteemed more or less sacred; the common people did not feed upon them and the priests never tasted them, because of their reputed sanctity, while at times they were worshiped as real deities. Cities were named after them and temples built to them. In different parts of Egypt different fish were worshiped individually; the Greek comedians even made fun of the Egyptians because of this fact. Dagon figures as the Fish-god, and the female deity known as Athor, in Egypt, is undoubtedly the same as Aphrodite of the Greeks and Venus of the Romans, who were believed to have sprung from the sea. Lucian tells us that this worship was of great antiquity; strange as this idolatry may appear, it was yet most wide-spread and included also the veneration which the Egyptians, before Moses, paid to the river Nile. It is important to remember that Nun, the name of the father of Joshua, is the Semitic word for fish, while the phallic character of the fish in Chaldean mythology cannot be gainsaid. Nim, the planet Saturn, was the fish-god of Berosus, and the same as the Assyrian god Asshur, whose name and office are strikingly similar to those of the Hebrew leader Joshua.

Corresponding to the ancient phallus or lingam, which was the masculine phallic symbol, we have the Kteis or Yoni as the symbol of the female principle; but an emblem of similar import is often to be met with in the shape of the shell, the fig leaf or the letter delta, as may be frequently seen from ancient coins and monuments. Similar attributes were at other times expressed by a bird, using the dove or sparrow, which will at once make one think of the prominence given to the dove in the fable of Noah and the Ark.

Referring again to the fish symbol let me say that the head of Proserpine is very often represented surrounded by dolphins; sometimes by pomegranates which also have a phallic significance. In fact, Inman in his work on Ancient Faiths says of the pomegranate, "The shape of this fruit much resembles that of the gravid uterus in the female, and the abundance of seeds which it contains makes it a fitting emblem of the prolific womb of the celestial mother. Its use was largely adopted In various forms of worship; It was united with bells in the adornment of the robes of the Jewish High Priest; it was introduced as an ornament into Solomon's Temple, where it was united with lilies and with the lotus."

Its arcane meaning is undoubtedly phallic. In fact, as Inman has stated, the idea of virility was most closely interwoven with religion, though the English Egyptologists have suppressed a portion of the facts in the history which they have given the world; but the practice which still obtains among certain Negroes of Northern Africa of mutilating every male captive and slain enemy is but a continuance of the practice alluded to in the 2nd Book of Kings, 20:18, Isaiah, 39:17, and 1st Samuel 18:26. Frequently in sacred Scripture we find allusions to the Pillar as a most sacred emblem, as for example in Isaiah 19-19, "In that day there shall be an altar to the Lord in the midst of the land of Egypt and a pillar to the border thereof to Jehovah," etc. Moreover God was supposed to have appeared to his chosen people as a pillar of fire. Nevertheless when among idolatrous nations pillars were set up as a part of their rites we find them noticed in Scripture as an abomination, as for example, Deut. 12:3, "Ye shall overthrow their altars and break their pillars;" Levit. 26:1, "Neither rear ye up a standing image."

THE EVIL EYE

Among the Jews the pillar had much the same significance as the pyramid among the Egyptians or the triangle or cone among votaries of other worships. The Tower of Babel must have been purely a mythical creation but in the same direction. Although Abraham is regarded as having emigrated from Chaldea in the character of a dissenter from the religion of his country (see Joshua 24:2-3), his immediate descendants apparently had recourse to the symbols to which I have alluded. Thus he erected altars and planted pillars wherever he resided, and conducted his son to the land of Moriah to sacrifice him to the deity, as was done among the Phoenicians. Jeptha in like manner sacrificed his own daughter Mizpeh, and the temple of Solomon was supposed to have been built upon the site of Abraham's ancient altar. Jacob not only set up a pillar at the place which he called Bethel but made libations; Samuel worshiped at the High Places at Ramah, and Solomon at the Great Stone in Gibeon. It remained for Hezekiah to change the entire Hebrew cult. He removed the Dionysiac statues and phallic pillars as well as the conical and omphalic symbols of Venus and Ashtaroth, broke in pieces the brazen serpent of Moses and overthrew the mounds and altars. After him Josiah removed the paraphernalia of sun worship and destroyed the statues and emblems of Venus and Adonis, (2nd Kings, 23:4-20).

The Greek Hermes was identical with the Egyptian Khem, as well as with Mercury and with Priapus, also with the Hebrew Eloah; thus when Jacob entered into a covenant with Laban his father-in-law, a pillar was set up and a heap of stones made and a certain compact entered into; similar land marks were usual with the Greeks and placed by them upon public roads. As Mrs. Childs has beautifully said, "Other emblems deemed sacred by Hindus and worshiped in their temples have brought upon them the charge of gross indecencies... The light with its grand revealings, and heat, making the earth fruitful with beauty, excited wonder and worship among the first inhabitants of our world, is it strange that they likewise regarded with reverence the great mystery of human birth? Were they impure thus to regard it? Or are we impure that we do not so regard it?"

Constant, in his work on Roman Polytheism says, "Indecent rites may be practiced by religious people with the greatest purity of heart, but when incredulity has gained a footing among these peoples then those rites become the cause and pretext of the most revolting corruption." The phallic symbol was always found in temples of Siva, who corresponds to Baal, and was usually placed as are the most precious emblems of our Christian temples today, in some inmost recess of the sanctuary. Moreover lamps with seven branches were kept burning before it, these seven branched lamps long antedating the golden candlestick of the Mosaic Tabernacle. The Jews by no means escaped the objective evidence of phallic worship; in Ezekiel 16:17, is a very marked allusion to the manufacture by Jewish women of gold and silver phalli.

As a purely phallic symbol and custom mark the significance of certain superstitions and practices even now prevalent in Great Britain. Thus in Boylase's History of Cornwall it is stated that there is a stone in the Parish of Mardon, with a hole in it fourteen inches in diameter, through which many persons creep for the relief of pains in the back and limbs, and through which children are drawn to cure them of rickets, this being a practical application of the doctrine of regeneration. In 1888 there was printed in The London Standard a considerable reference to passing children through clefts in trees as a curative measure for certain physical ailments. The same practice prevails in Brazil and in many other places, and with the present generation it has been customary to split young ash tree and, opening this, pass through it a child for the purpose of curing rupture or some other bodily ailment.

The phallic element most certainly cannot be denied in Christianity itself, since in it are many references which to the initiated are unmistakable. From the fall of man with its serpent myth and its phallic foundation to the peculiar position assigned to the Virgin Mary as a mother, phallic references abound. However, it should not be forgotten that whatever were the primitive ideas on which these dogmas were based, they had been lost sight of or had been received in a fresh aspect by the founders of Christianity. The fish and the cross originally typified the idea of generation and later that of life, in which sense they were applied to Christ. The most plainly phallic representation used in early Christian Iconography, is undoubtedly the Aureole or elliptical framework, containing usually the figure of Christ, sometimes that of Mary. The Nimbus also, generally circular but sometimes triangular, is of positive phallic significance, even though it contain within it the name of Jehovah. The sun flowers which sometimes are made to surround the figure of St. John the Evangelist are the lotus flowers of the Egyptians. The divine hand with the thumb and two fingers outstretched, even though it rests on a cruciform nimbus, is a phallic emblem, and is used by the Neapolitans of today to avert the Evil Eye, although it was originally a symbol of Isis. Indeed the Virgin Mary is the ancient Isis, as can be most easily established, since the virgin "Succeeded to her form, titles, symbols, rites and ceremonies." (King). The great image still moves in procession as when Juvenal laughed at it, and her proper title is the exact translation of the Sanskrit and the equivalent of the modern Madonna, the Lotus of Isis, and the Lily of the modern Mary. Indeed, as King has written, "It is astonishing how much of the Egyptian symbolism passed over into usages of the following times." The high cap and hooked staff of the god became the bishop's miter and crozier. The term Nun is purely Egyptian and bore its present meaning. The Crux Ansata, testifying the union of the male and female principle in the most obvious manner, and denoting fecundity and abundance, is transformed by a simple inversion into an orb surmounted by a cross, the ensign of royalty.

The teaching of the Church of Rome regarding the Virgin Mary shows a remarkable resemblance to the teachings of the ancients concerning the female associate of the triune deity.

THE EVIL EYE

In ancient times she has passed under many and diverse names; she was the Virgin, conceiving and bringing forth from her own inherent power; she was the wife of Nimrod; she has been known as Athor, Artemis, Aphrodite, Venus, Isis, Cybele, etc.

As Anaitis she is Mother and Child, appearing again as Isis and Horus; even in ancient Mexico Mother and Child were worshiped. In modern times she reappears as the Virgin Mary and her Son; she was queen of fecundity, queen of the gods, goddess of war. Virgin of the Zodiac, the mysterious Virgin "Time" from whose womb all things were born. Although variously represented she has been usually pictured as a more or less nude figure carrying an infant in her arms. (Inman, "Ancient Faiths").

Inman declares without hesitation that the trinity of the ancients is unquestionably of phallic origin, and others have strenuously contended and apparently proven that the male emblem of generation in divine creation was three in one, and that the female emblem has always been the triangle or accepted symbol of trinity. Sometimes two triangles have been combined forming a six-rayed star, the two together being emblematic of the union of the male and female principles producing a new figure; the triangle by itself with the point down typifies the delta or yoni through which all things come Into the world. Another symbol of deity among the Indians was the Trident, and this marks the belief in the Trinity which very generally prevailed in India among the Hindus. As Maurice says, "It was indeed highly proper and strictly characteristic that a three-fold deity should wield a triple scepter." Upon the top of the immense pyramids of Deoghur, which were truncated, and upon whose upper surface rested the circular cone- that ancient emblem of the Phallus and of the Sun, was found the trident scepter of the Greek Neptune. It is said that in India is to be found the most ancient form of Trinitarian worship. In Egypt it later prevailed widely, but scarcely any two states worshiped the same triad, though all triads had this in common at least that they were father, mother and son, or male and female with their progeny. In the course of time, however, the worship of the first person was lost or absorbed in the second and the same thing is prevalent among the Christians of today, for many churches and institutions are dedicated to the second or third persons of the Trinity but none to the first.

The transition from the old to the new could not be effected in a short time and must have been an exceedingly slow process, therefore we need not be surprised to be told of the ancient worship that after Its exclusion from larger places it was maintained for a long time by the inhabitants of humbler localities; hence its subsequent designation, since from being kept up in the villages, the pagi, its votaries, were designated pagani, or pagans. Even now some of these ancient superstitions remain in recognizable form. The moon is supposed to exert a baneful or lucky influence according as it is first viewed; the mystic horse-shoe, which is a purely uterine symbol, is still widely employed; lucky and unlucky days are still regarded; our playing cards are indicated by phallic symbols, the spade, the triadic club, the omphallic distaff and eminence disguised as the heart and the diamonds. Dionysius reappears as St. Denys, or in France as St. Bacchus; Satan is revered as St. Satur or St. Swithin; the Holy Virgin, Astraea, whose return was heralded by Virgil as introducing the Golden Age, is now designated as the Blessed Virgin, Queen of Heaven. The Mother and Child are today in Catholic countries adored as much as were Ceres and Bacchus, or Isis and the infant Horus, centuries ago. The nuns of Christian today are the nuns of the Buddhists or of the Egyptian worshipers of Isis, and the phallic import is not lost even in their case since they are the "Brides of the Savior." The libations of human blood which were formerly offered to Bacchus found most tragic imitation in the sacrifices of later days. The screechings of the ancient prophets of Baal, and of the Egyptian worshipers, preceded the flagellations of the penitents. Even recently, during Holy Week in Rome, devotees lash themselves until the blood runs, as did the young men in ancient Rome during the Lupercalia. And even yet in New Mexico the Indian penitents repeat the cruel flagellations and cross-bearing taught by the Spanish priest, to the extent- sometimes- of an actual crucifixion. In the ancient Roman catacombs are found portraits of the utensils and furniture of the ancient mysteries, and one drawing shows a woman standing before an altar offering buns to a certain god. In fact we may say there is no Christian fast nor festival, procession nor sacrament, custom nor example, that do not come quite naturally from previous paganism. The Creation is in fact a human rather than a divine product, in this sense that it was suggested to the mind of man by the existence of things, while its method was, at least at first, suggested by the operations of nature; thus man saw the living bird emerge from the egg, after a certain period of incubation, a phenomenon equivalent to actual creation as apprehended by his simple mind. Incubation obviously then associated itself with Creation, and this fact will explain the universality with which the egg was received as a symbol in the earlier systems of cosmogony. By a similar process creation came to be symbolized in the form of a phallus, and so the Egyptians, in their refinement of these ideas, adopted as their symbol of the first great cause, a Scarabaeus, indicating the great hermaphroditic unity since they believed this insect to be both male and female.

Further exemplification of the same underlying principle is seen in the fact that most all of the ancient deities were paired, thus we have heaven and earth, sun and moon, fire and earth, father and mother, etc. Faber says- "The Ancient Pagans of almost every part of the globe were wont to symbolize the world by an egg; hence this symbol is introduced into the cosmogonies of nearly all nations, and there are few persons even among those who have made mythology their study to whom the mundane egg is not perfectly familiar; it is the emblem not only of earth and life but also of the universe in its largest extent."

I began this essay with the intention of demonstrating the recondite but positive connection between the symbolism of the

Church of today and the phallic and iatric cults of pre-christian centuries. (Much of the subject matter contained in the previous essay (III) may be profitably read in this connection) As a humble disciple of that Aesculapius who was the reputed founder of our craft, I have felt that every genuine scholar in medicine should be familiar with these relations between the past and the present.

V: THE RELATION OF THE GRECIAN MYSTERIES TO THE FOUNDATION OF CHRISTIANITY

Ever since mentality has been an attribute of mankind, man has appreciated that he is surrounded by a vast incomprehensible mystery which ever closes in upon him, and from whose environment he may never free himself. The endeavor to solve this mystery has on one hand stimulated his reasoning power, and on the other nearly paralyzed it. Having no better guidance he has in all time attributed to a Great First Cause powers and faculties, even shape and form, more or less human; thus from time immemorial God or the Gods have been given a kingdom, a throne, some definite form, and even offspring. To him or them have been given purely human attributes, and they have been supposed to possess human passions and to be capable of love, wrath, strength, etc. In nearly all ages lightning, for instance, has been regarded as an expression of divine fury. As intelligence advanced the number of Gods was reduced and their manifestations classified and studied more or less imaginatively; and so while men have always acknowledged the impossibility of explaining the great mysteries of creation and of space, they have seemed to find it necessary to create other equally inscrutable mysteries of purely human invention, such as the incarnation, the trinity, the resurrection, vicarious salvation, metempsychosis, and the like.

History shows the love of mystery to be contagious as well as productive of its kind, and the origin of mystic teachings as well as of most secret societies bears out these statements. Secrets, guarded by fearful oaths, personified by meaningless emblems, concealed either in language unintelligible to others, or else hidden in terms whose special meaning is known only to the initiated, made attractive by special signs, symbols, innocent rites, or barbarous observances- all of these means were designed solely to keep men banded together for the purpose of forming a propaganda intended to perpetuate yet other mysteries in which the initiates were especially interested. Since history began such associations of men have existed for most diverse ends, all having this in common, that only by this means could they secure and maintain influence and power. And so the series of pictures which represent man in this role may be regarded as a panorama, led by garlanded priests carrying images of Isis or droning hymns to Demeter of Eleusis, or Druids preparing for their human sacrifices; followed by gay and voluptuous Bacchantes, succeeded by white-robed Pythagoreans; next may come the suffering Essenes bearing crosses, then the Latin Brotherhoods, followed by the German and English Guilds, the Stone Masons with their Implements, the Crusader Knights, those coming first having an appearance of actual humility and devotion, while those who follow are haughty and contemptuous to a degree. Then would follow the black-robed Penitents and the members of the Society of Jesus, sanctimonious, with eyes cast down, human machines, mere tools in the hands of their superiors; the panorama continuing with a widely assorted lot of scholars, artisans and men of all conditions in various regalia, and terminated with an indistinguishable multitude of variously adorned men, some sleek and fat, others ill-conditioned, some devout and sincere, others mere jesters and knaves from every walk of life.

It was most natural and to be expected that primitive man should be most profoundly Impressed with the forces of nature, often terrifying and frightful, often winsome and attractive, and that he should bow himself down to the unknown cause of these manifestations. With his extremely finite mind he necessarily personified them; after having done this he proceeded to propitiate them by worship with certain forms of ritual. Perhaps fire first and most of all attracted him in this way, and drew from him the earliest acts of worship, for in spite of the general views to the contrary fire is often of natural origin, and must have been known to men before they became able to produce it by their own efforts. From practical to generalized concepts was a natural step, and thus mythology had its beginnings; the earliest distinctions were as between that which is overhead, i. e. Heaven, and that which is beneath, namely, the earth; these are the beginnings of all cosmogonies. Next the Gods were given the attributes of sex; Heaven was represented as masculine, fructifying, powerful; Earth as conceptive, female and gentle. By the union of these two were produced sun, moon and their progeny- the stars. Later the sun became Poseidon or Neptune, because he appeared from and disappeared into the sea. Then the imagination began to run riot, and gave rise to many individual divinities, gods and goddesses, all with human passions and attributes, mingling and propagating after human fashion, and begetting dynasties and half human races, whose doings were the subject of countless epics, dramas, myths and romances.

Thus time passed on and the original sense or meaning of these myths, descending slowly by oral tradition, became lost, while the myths themselves were for a long time accepted as historical facts. Nevertheless in all ages there have been men who, like Aristotle, Cicero and Plutarch, have questioned the accuracy of these statements and shown themselves intelligent and active skeptics. During all these times, however, a wily priest-craft had lived and thrived on the superstitions of the common people and the practices in which they have indulged; by these men, thus conditioned, any active doubt was regarded as subversive of the system by which they were supported, and as one not to be tolerated- this condition pertaining not only to antiquity, since it is too significant a feature even of the early years of this twentieth century. A more or less honest though misinformed priesthood has, in all times, been in favor of the purification of the theology in vogue in their times and among their inner circles, and has in the main given the most rationalistic interpretation to the obscure things which they taught, and practiced what their education and environment would permit. But in order to preserve the mysteries, to maintain them as such, and save themselves from becoming superfluous, not to say intolerable, these same mysteries have been tricked out with mysticism, symbolism of the most fantastic character, and allegory of the most bewildering kind; moreover this has often been accomplished by dramatic representations and by moralizing or demoralizing ceremonies. The countries in which these "mysteries," as they have since been known, were most commonly practiced and most widely believed were Egypt, Chaldea and Greece.

The sources of the Egyptian mysteries, like those of Egyptian civilization, are the most difficult to discover. The Nile is necessarily the basis of Egyptian history, geography, activity and habits, and consequently must be also of the Egyptian cult. The people who were known as Egyptians invaded the land of the Nile from the direction of Asia, and found there a race of negro type whom they subdued and with whom they later mingled. The Semites called the land Misraim; the Greeks finally changed the name of its great river to Neilos. The country is a land of enigmas. Who built those pyramids, and why? Who originated the system of pictorial writing which we call the hieroglyphic? Who planned those wonderful temples now either in ruins, as in upper Egypt, or buried beneath the desert sands, as in lower Egypt? Who brought and erected those mighty blocks of stone or massive slabs from enormous distances, and handled them as we could scarcely do today with the best of modern machinery?

In course of time two hereditary classes were formed, the priests who dominated the minds, and the warriors who controlled the bodies of the conquered people and the lower classes. The latter kept the throne of Egypt occupied, while the former, having a monopoly of the knowledge of the time, prescribed for the people what they must believe, yet were very far from accepting these precepts for themselves, and in their inner circles made light of that which they preached to the despised classes without. The Egyptians named their Sun God RA, but assigned the various attributes of the sun to different personalities; they had moreover not only Gods for the whole land, but Ptah was God of Memphis, Ammon God of Thebes, etc. Local deities were often constructed out of inspiring objects or from animals inhabited by spirits, and thus the fetishism of the original negro race exerted no little influence upon the higher cult of their lighter colored conquerors. Worship was paid to animals not for their own sake but because of the Gods who were supposed to reside within them; thus their prominent Gods were represented with the head of some animal. This honor belonged not to any individual animal but of necessity to the entire species, certain representatives of which were maintained at public expense in the temples, where they were carefully guarded and waited upon by the faithful. To harm one of these animals was to be severely punished, to kill one of them was to die. Conversely when a God failed in responding to the prayers of the faithful his fetish had to suffer, and the priests first threatened the animal, and if menaces were unavailing they killed the sacred beast, albeit in secret, lest the people should learn of it.

As time went on there was less of zoolatry, and the Sun-Gods and their associates figured more largely among the cult of the people. The sun's course was not represented as that of a chariot, as among the Persians and Greeks, but rather as the voyage of a Nile boat, upon which the God Re navigated the heavens; from which it will appear that the priestly religion was making slow progress to monotheism by means of oligotheism. The secret teaching of the priests was now more and more to the effect that the Gods stood not so much for themselves as for something else. During the fourth dynasty the lower Egyptian city Anu was known as the City of the Sun, hence the Greek name for the place, Heliopolis. Still more characteristic was the giving of the name of Osiris, who figured as God of Abdu, which the Greeks called Abydos, in upper Egypt, to the God of the Sunset, who was king of the lower domains and of death, brother and at the same time husband of Isis, brother also of Set, who slew him, and father of Horus, i. e. God of the new sun, who figures after each sunset. Horus fought with Set, but being unable to completely destroy him left him the desert as his kingdom, while himself holding to the Nile valley.

This story of the Gods was publicly represented in various scenes on certain holidays, but only the priests, i. e., the initiated, knew the real meaning of the representations. Even the name of Osiris and his abode were kept secret, and outsiders heard only of the "great God" dwelling somewhere in "the West." These were the most famous of all the old Egyptian mysteries, though to them were added many others, including that of Apis, the sacred bull of Memphis, who served also as the symbol of the Sun and of the fructifying Nile; beneath his tongue was to be seen the sacred beetle, and the behavior of the great animal was supposed to be prophetic and his actions to mean oracular sayings. The Sphinx again was a sun-God, his image being repeated throughout the Nile region, and was always thought of as a male; the head was represented as that of some king, while the whole figure stood for the Sun-God Harmachis; although the sphinx later introduced into Greece was always female.

While the Egyptians did not attribute to their numerous Gods divine perfection, they nevertheless regarded religious practices as a means of currying favor with their divinities, a custom apparently still in favor. The priests believed in a Sun-God as the only true deity, but not so the people; thus the priests in the various cities praised their local and tutelary God as supreme and made him identical with Re, whose name they appended to the original, as for instance Amon-Re. The king, no matter where he was, prayed always to the local deity as lord of heaven and earth, yet in words always the same. At last during the eighteenth dynasty, about 1460 B. C, Amenhotep IV realized that the power of the priesthood was a menace to the crown and therefore proclaimed the Sun as the sole God, not in human shape, but in that of a disk. He ordered all other images of other Gods associated with the sun to be destroyed; the priests of these deposed Gods lost their places and estates, which latter were confiscated. But his sons-in-law who succeeded him restored the deposed monarchs. Nevertheless they were marked as heretics by those priests who were reinstated in their former power. In consequence of this conflict, which was violent and prolonged, the intellectual life of Egypt was paralyzed and the mystic teachings of the priests were henceforth not disturbed by any wave of progress or advance.

The people again sank into a stupid and unredeemable formalism, demonism and sorcery. With the purpose of amusing them the priests furnished gorgeous sacrificial processions and festivals, while at the same time drawing them away from the true God by teaching them a worship of deceased kings and queens. They also built temples, to only the outer portion of which were the people generally admitted, while the innermost portions were guarded by these priests lest the mysteries thus protected be such no longer. They also procured the building of the ancient Labyrinth, near Lake Moeris, of which Herodotus tells us that there were fifteen hundred chambers above ground and as many more under ground, which latter were never shown except to the initiated, and which contained the remains of sacred crocodiles and of the Pharaohs.

The Egyptian priests taught that man was made up of body, a material essence or the soul, which in the shape of a bird left the body at death, and an immaterial spirit which held to the man the same relation which a God held to the animal in which he dwelt, and which at death departed from the body like the image of a dream. They taught also that, if the soul and spirit were to live on, the body should be embalmed and laid in a rock chamber, and that then the relatives must supply meat, drink, and clothing for its use. The spirit took its way to Osiris and by means of a magic formula the dead would be made one with Osiris; hence in the Egyptian "Book of the Dead" the deceased was addressed as Osiris with his own name added, and could now lead a happy life in the other world, which life was portrayed on the walls of the Sepulchers in pictures which are still to be seen, showing how the creature comforts of this world were to be enhanced in the next. Having reached the outer world, and having escaped the host of demons that threatened him on his passage, he could then revisit this earth at will in any form.

The Egyptian priests also taught that there was a judgment of the dead, and that new comers had to appear before Osiris, with his forty-two Assessors, and disclaim the commission of each one of forty-two sins; all of which was a magic formula for obtaining bliss according to their notion rather than anything intended as a true statement. The hippopotamus figured as an active agent in the Book of the Dead, appearing always as the accuser, when the sins and the good deeds were being weighed in the balance, while the God Thoth was the "attorney for the defense." All these secret doctrines of a priestcraft necessitated secret associations, at least of the higher priests, to which the king was always admitted, the only Egyptian outside of the priesthood to be thus taught their secrets. This was purely for protection; having less fear of foreigners these priests often initiated distinguished men from foreign lands, Greeks especially. Thus Orpheus, Homer, Lycurgus, Solon, Herodotus, Pythagoras, Plato, Archimedes, and many others, received the secret doctrine. The ritual was a long and tedious but significant ceremony, taught by degrees like the Masonry of today, and necessitated in some cases the right of circumcision; all who passed it were pledged to the most strict silence. According to Diodorus the Orphic Mysteries were in large degree a repetition of the Egyptian, while the Greek legislators, philosophers and mathematicians whom I have named drew their knowledge from the same source; all of which is probably a very gross exaggeration.

Nevertheless it would appear from the hieroglyphic remains that high grade schools were conducted by the Egyptian priests, and that foreign scholars could obtain for themselves instruction in the exact sciences of the day. Only the priests, however, were able to write the hieroglyphics, at least in the earlier centuries of Egyptian history. There can be no doubt but that the secret doctrine of the Egyptian priests was both philosophical and religious, and was sharply distinguished from the popular belief which mistook tradition for truth; that it was monotheistic, that it rejected polytheism and zoolatry, and that the true signification of Egyptian mythology was expounded in private. Moreover an essential part of this mystery concerned the interpretation of myths as allegorical accounts of personified natural phenomena. For instance Plutarch ("Isis and Osiris") writes- "When we hear of the Egyptian myths of the Gods, their wanderings, their dismemberment and other like incidents, we must recall the remarks already made, so as to understand that the stories told are not to be taken literally as recounting actual occurrences."

Without now going into the subject of the relative age of the Egyptian and Chaldean cults, I will remind you that the secret wisdom of one race was not excelled by that of the other. The Chaldean races are undoubtedly of Turanian origin, and their form of religion was peculiar to the Ural-Altaic stock and the Turkic races, who originated the Cuneiform writing. Their most ancient writings represented evil spirits as coming from the desert in groups of seven, and contained formulas for exorcising them; they were presided over by the heavens, while from the higher spirits evolved Gods and Goddesses in countless number. Upon the original ground work of Chaldean ideas a Semitic race built a superstructure, and the first traces of the Babylonians and Assyrians appeared some four thousand years B. C. Their highest God was an individual whom they named Baal, while the sun and moon were his images. As in Egypt the priests were held in great reverence, standing next after the king, who was *ex officio* high priest; they too had a secret doctrine withheld from the vulgar. Although the Chaldeans were astrologers rather than astronomers, they were yet familiar enough with the heavens to estimate astral phenomena for what they really were, instead of holding them to be Gods, though they may have represented them as such to the common people. Their literature contained numerous mythological poems, so obscure that to understand them a key was required, which key was only in the possession of the priests. Inasmuch as Abraham came from Ur in Chaldea, with him crept into biblical literature much of the Chaldean tradition and folklore. The Chaldeans had also their Noah, and their deluge, in which the dove figured as in the biblical account. When the proprietor of the Ark finally freed the animals he erected an altar and offered sacrifice, to which the Gods gathered "like masses of flies." This story contributes but one section of the great Chaldean epic in which are recounted the exploits of a hero corresponding with the Nimrod of the Hebrew Bible, dating from the twenty-third century B. C, and reminding one forcibly of the Herculean and many other myths recounted in other ancient languages.

An off-shoot of the Chaldean culture was that of Persia, whose priestly class were far removed above the warriors and farmers that constituted the other two classes. Priests married only among their own race, possessed all the knowledge, made their king *ex oficio* one of themselves, and practiced itinerant teaching, but solely among their own caste. In the holy city, Ragha, the priests alone held rule and no secular power prevailed; Zoroaster was their founder; they were the physicians, astrologers, interpreters of dreams, scribes and officers of justice, while they impressed upon the minds of the people their exclusive duties- to reverence the holy fire, which was their greatest mystery, to listen to the teaching of passages from the sacred book, and to perform numerous ceremonies of purification. Only the initiated were taught the meaning of the strife between the good Ormuzd and the evil Ahriman, which was probably the alternation of day and night, and of summer and winter. In India the intense feeling with regard to caste but little altered the condition of things from that obtaining as above described, though the Brahmins were further away from the other castes than in other countries where the priests came from the common people; by the latter the Brahmins used to be regarded as Gods and did all they could to perpetuate this feeling. By this fact alone they became a self-constituted mystic organization, being themselves pantheists while the people were idolaters. Though they taught pantheism in their sacred books, the second and third castes, namely the warriors and farmers, did not understand the teaching, and the fourth caste dared not read them at all.

In this pantheism penitents and hermits were esteemed as above kings and heroes; but even the life of a hermit was not exacting enough for them, so they organized the idea of a soul of the universe so incomprehensible that, as they themselves acknowledged, no man could comprehend it or instruct another in it. Despairing of solving the problem they finally fancied that the universe was a phantasm, and that the earth and all things earthly were nothing. They taught that through countless aeons of time men grew always worse, and were born only to suffer and die, or to do penance in the torments of an indescribable Hell. Naturally of all these things the people could only understand the teachings pertaining to Hell and future punishment, and so the Brahmins contrived for them a supreme deity, having the same name as their Soul of the Universe, namely Brahma, whom they made the creator but playing a passive part. The people were not content, however, with an absentee passive God, but paid much more attention to Vishnu the preserver, and the dreaded Siva, the destroyer.

After a while these three Gods were united in a sort of trinity, represented by a three headed figure, but without temples or sacrifices. The Brahmins continued their subtleties and divided the people into parties, like the scholiasts and disputants of the middle centuries of our present Christian era, and so the Hindu religion became more and more debased. However, in the sixth century B. C, Buddha, that great figure in early history, endeavored to save it by a reform which found much more encouragement in the West, and to the far East of India, than in India Itself, and which has since assumed a more composite character by fusion with the religions of the surrounding countries. Buddha formed first a monastic society based upon ethical doctrines, whose underlying principle was that only by a renunciation of everything can man find safety, peace and comfort. Buddha's first teachings were mystic and for the initiated only; his followers believed also in reincarnation. After his death and that of those who were supposed to have lived before him, and who were expected to appear again, and who had been raised to the dignity of Gods, (and after their number had been added to that of the popular Hindu Gods and to the Gods of the other people), then Buddhism became a polytheism, and because of the variety of possible explanations and the necessary exegesis, assumed in the end the dimensions of a secret mystic doctrine.

The Hellenes undoubtedly did, in the beginning, worship natural forces under the form of animals, especially of serpents; later human and animal forms were united, and so they had deities with heads of animals, or with the bodies of horses like the Centaurs, or with the hoofs of goats like the Satyrs. But the natural Greek taste for the beautiful early asserted itself; the figures of Gods came by degrees to express the ideal of physical perfection, that is the human shape, and the Grecian religion became essentially a worship of the beautiful, and not as among Oriental religions a worship of the unnatural or hideous. They forgot the astronomic and cosmic significance of the early myths and held rather to personifications of the normal forces, of which their poets sang as of mortal heroes. They never dreamed of dogma, creed or revelation, demanded only that man honor the Gods, but left it to the taste of each one how he should suitably perform his acts of reverence.

It must be confessed, however, that in candor and chastity they left much to be desired; but this may be explained when we remember that their own Gods set them a very poor example in these respects. Still history will forgive them much because they loved much. The Greeks were exceedingly liberal in their interpretations concerning the Gods, while the various peoples constituting the Greek race were not at all agreed as to the number and respective rank of the Gods whom they worshiped. Thus one would be disowned here, another there; while in one place greater honor would be paid to one, or elsewhere to another; exactly as in the case of the Saints among the Catholic people of today. They went so far in their worship of the beautiful as to divide the Gods among the localities which possessed statues of them, which Gods came to be regarded as distinct individuals; so that even Socrates doubted whether Aphrodite of the sky and Aphrodite of the people were or were not the same person. Furthermore in their liberality they made Gods to hand for every emergency, and even worshiped the unknown Gods, as St. Paul long ago recorded. For the Greeks these Gods were neither monsters like those of Egypt, India and Chaldea, nor incorporeal spirits like the Gods of Persia and of Israel, but human beings with all the human attributes. For the Greeks neither Jehovah existed, nor a personal devil in any form.

Like the Greeks themselves their Gods had many human failings, though in them religion survived many mythological creations like the Centaurs, the Satyrs, etc. These were merely folklore beings enacting parts ranging from terror to farce, and never receiving divine honors. Grecian religion was, so to speak, the established church of the Greek states, but came to be in time a cloak for the designs of the politicians; in which respect history has many times repeated itself. For instance Socrates was made to drink his cup of hemlock on the pretext that he had apostatized from the state religion. Still even in his day heresy played no part except among politicians. Every one could plainly state his convictions, and Aristophanes in his comedies introduced Gods in the most ridiculous and compromising situations. So long as the public worship of the Gods went on the state cared little for the upholding of positive or suppressing of negative beliefs. The Gods were entitled to sacrifices and the people to divine aid, but they could regulate the interchange to suit themselves. The greatest public crimes were violation of temples and profanation of sacred things; one must leave the images alone even if he did not believe in the Gods they represented. Punishment of blasphemy was only inflicted when complaint was made. Foreign Gods could be introduced and worshiped at will, providing only that the customary honors were rendered to those at home.

Such religious freedom could naturally only exist during the minority or the absence of a priestly class. Anyone could transact business with the Gods or conduct sacrifices; priests were employed only in the temples, and outside of them they had neither business, influence nor privileges. Their pantheism was comprehensive; the Gods were everywhere, and the honor done to them consisted in invocations, votive offerings and sacrifices. The Grecian religion recognized no official revelation which all were required to believe, though it did not deny the possibility of revelations at any time. Their oracles were obtainable only in particular places and through duly qualified individuals. At one time in ancient Greece conjuration was in vogue, but the Gods and demons who indulged in it were all borrowed from foreign sources, and in time it degenerated into pure magic.

The Greeks, however, could not get away from the sentimental notion that belief in the Gods must have an ethical side and must be subordinate to their faith; in other words that human nature was something entirely different from the divine to which it was subject. Alienation from the God in which they believed led necessarily to the impulse to seek him, which was the leading motive in the institution of the Grecian mysteries-Gods who were man's equals were not sufficient for the Greeks. In the beginning of these mysteries they borrowed the art of the popular religion, disregarded the science of the day as well as the philosophic doctrines of their great men, held in contempt both human power and human knowledge, and devoted themselves almost entirely to self-introspection, meditation on revelation, incarnation and resurrection, and presented these things in dramatic forms and ceremonies, by which illusions they hoped to make more or less impression upon the senses. The

THE EVIL EYE

Grecian mysteries were the opposite of genuine Hellenism. The true Greek was cheerful, happy, clear in perception, and his Gods appeared to him as do their statues to us today. But Greek mysticism was full of gloom, symbolism and fantastic interpretations; in every way it was unhellenic and abnormal, having no fit place in their soil nor in their age. It always has been the case that sentimental, romantic or mystical dispositions find delight in the mysterious, while logical minds are unmoved by it. From the Mysteries no man was excluded, save those who had shown themselves unworthy of Initiation. They had their origin in the early rites of purification and atonement; the former being at first only bodily cleansing, which later took on a moral significance; while the atonement was a sort of expiation which came with the consciousness of sin and desire for forgiveness.

Atonement was most called for in case of blood guiltiness, and consisted largely in the sacrifices of animals, burning of Incense, etc. In all the ancient mysteries these two features of purification and expiation played a great part. Of them all the oldest and most celebrated were those instituted at Eleusis, in Attica, in honor of the Goddess Demeter (Latin Ceres), and her daughter Persephone (Latin Proserpina). To these were added later a masculine deity, known at first as Iacchos, whose name is probably related to Jao, which appears in Jovispater or Jupiter, and to the Hebrew Yahve or Jehovah. Later, however, B was substituted for I and Iacchos was made to read Bacchus. Jao was the Harvest God, and consequently God of the grape, hence the close relation to Bacchus. The Greek word Eleusis means advent, and commemorates the visit of Demeter while wandering in search of her daughter- which reminds one of the Egyptian story of Isis. Moved by gratitude, Demeter bestowed upon the people of Eleusis the bread-grain and the mysteries. From this city the cult of these two deities spread over all Greece and most of Asia Minor, passed into Italy in modified form, and thus became widely accepted. The people built at Eleusis a temple in pure Doric style and a Mystic House in which the secret festivals were held. The city was connected with

THE EVIL EYE

Athens by a Sacred Way, which was flanked with temples and sanctuaries, while in Athens itself was a building, the Eleusinion, in which a portion of the mysteries were celebrated. The buildings at Eleusis were in good preservation until the fourth century A. D., when they were destroyed by the Goths under Alaric, and at the instigation of monkish fanatics. You will see, then, that the mysteries were widely observed in Asia Minor, and at a time when they must have deeply tinged the religious views and habits of a large portion of the population prior to the beginning of the Christian Era.

The Eleusinian mysteries were always under the direction of the Athenian government, and the report of their celebration was always rendered to the grand council of Athens. The function of the priests was an hereditary and exclusive privilege and the mysteries as a whole were under the immediate care of a sacred council. The people contented themselves mainly with honoring the Gods, while in these mysteries the original endeavor was to emphasize the preeminence of the divine over the human, hence their careful guardianship by the authorities of the state. Both were offshoots of pantheism, one seeing the divine in all earthly things, the other constantly searching for it there, and striving to unite with it. Monotheism, that is absolute separation of the human from the divine without hope of union, is a purely Oriental conception, quite incomprehensible to the Greek mind. No ancient Greek ever conceived of a creative deity in the Egyptians' sense, nor of a vengeful Jehovah like that of the Hebrews. The Eleusinian mysteries were most highly venerated among the Greeks; so much so that during their celebration hostilities were suspended between opposing armies, while those who witnessed them uninvited or betrayed the secret teaching, or ridiculed them, were executed or banished. So late even as the period of the Roman supremacy the Roman Emperors took an interest in maintaining these mysteries, and some of the early Christian Emperors, like Constantius II. and Jovian, while forbidding nocturnal festivals made an exception of these.

THE EVIL EYE

The sum of the original Eleusinian doctrine is a myth based upon the rape of Demeter's daughter Persephone by Pluto, all of which is the old story of the seasons and the changes brought about in their regular succession; and as Persephone was ultimately united with Bacchus but returned to the lower world for the winter, we see typified first, the fruitfulness of the Sun God; secondly, the fecundity of the soil, and, thirdly, the resurrection of the body, which having been dropped like the grain into the earth was supposed to rise from it again after a similar fashion. How much this may have to do with present Christian beliefs concerning the resurrection may not be easily decided. Nevertheless it is of interest that the doctrine of the resurrection is of pre-Christian origin and is traceable through heathen teachings, even if having no greater support than the analogy above cited. The central teaching of the mysteries was probably that of a personal immortality analogous to the return of bloom and blossom to plants in the spring. There were two festivals held at Eleusis, the lesser in March, when the ravished Persephone came up out of the nether world into the sunlight; and the greater in October when she had to follow her sullen spouse into Hades again. The preliminary celebration was held at Athens, and lasted six days, from October 15th to 20th. They all assembled upon that day and went down to the seashore for the rite of purification, the other days being spent in sacrificing and marching in solemn procession. On the last of them came the grand Bacchic procession, when thousands of both sexes wended their way along the sacred road to Eleusis; the distance to be traveled was fourteen miles, but many stops were made. Arrived at Eleusis the first evening was devoted to drinking the decoction called kykeon, by which Demeter was originally comforted during her wanderings. During the first days the initiated feasted and performed their mystic rites, consisting largely of torch light processions at night. After these were over the festival became a scene of merriment and athletic competition.

The fasting and solemn cup, along with others of their rites, remind one of certain Christian observations perpetuated to the present day, while the severe tests to which those desiring initiation were subject have been more or less imitated by the Free Masons and other secret societies of medieval or modern times. The Mystic House must have been furnished with all the resources of the stage and the most ingenious stage carpentry of that day, and makes one think of Scottish Rite Masonry of this. The initiates regarded their chances in the next world as much better than those of the common people, as all the ancient Greek writers acknowledge.

In age and renown the mysteries of the Cabiri, in the island of Samothrace, rank next to those of Eleusis. They date back to a time preceding the evolution of several of the Grecian deities. These Mysteries implied originally an astro-mythology, losing in time its astral meaning. In these Samothracian mysteries the reproductive forces of nature figured most prominently, and through them the Phallic worship of the Orientals was transmitted to the Greeks. Into these mysteries women and even children were initiated. There were also Cabirian mysteries In several other islands in the Grecian Archipelago, as well as on the continent. Mysteries were also celebrated in the Island of Crete, in honor of Zeus. We know but little concerning them save that in the spring time the birth of the God was commemorated in one place, and his death at another, and that amid loud noises the story of the childhood of Zeus was enacted by the young. As already remarked the worship of Bacchus was imported and in him was personified the influence of the sun upon the growth of the vine, while the ultimate tendency was to the glorification of life and force; in other words, it was eminently materialistic and appealed to the grosser senses. The Dionysian mysteries originated in Thrace, and among a people of Pelasgian stock, who were naturally gloomy save when aroused, when their enthusiasm became exaggerated into transports of frenzy. In time a distinction obtained between the Dionysian mysteries and the festivals. At least seven different non-mystic festivals occurred in Attica during the year, which were of popular character, during which the Phallic worship, if any, predominated. The fabled adventures of Bacchus were enacted and the dramatic stage originated at this time and from this beginning. On the other hand, a triennial festival of Dionysos was held in which women participated who, saturated with wine, lost all restraint and humility and were called maenades or mad women, while their festivals were spoken of as orgia, whence our modern term orgies.

These were conducted at night, upon the mountains, by torch-light, in mid-winter, while the women, who were clothed in skins, shunned all association with men, and drank, danced, sang and committed all sorts of excesses, finally sacrificing a bull, in honor of the god, whose flesh they devoured raw. They then raved about the death of their god and how he must be found again; all hope in rediscovering him centering in the quickening springtime. Bacchus worship, bad as it was in Greece, was surpassed in Rome, Livy even comparing the introduction of the Bacchic cult into Rome to a visitation of the plague. In its Etruscan and Roman form it became simple debauchery with a thin veneering of religion. So abominable did it become in time that in 186 B. C, the Consul Albinus was compelled to suppress it. Seven thousand persons were implicated at that time, and the ringleaders and a multitude of their accomplices were condemned to death or exile. The senate decreed that the Bacchanalia should never again be held in Rome or Italy, and the places sacred to Bacchic worship were to be destroyed. These orgies continued unchecked outside of Italy, and in time reappeared again even upon Italian soil, until the days of the Roman Emperors, when they reached a pitch of absolute shamelessness, as in the case of the notorious Messalina.

Time fails in which to mention all of the other debased mysteries which were met with in the various parts of Greece and Italy. Among them, however, must be recorded those of the mother of Rhea, those of Sebazios, and those of Mithras, all of which were finally collected by the sect of Orpheans. Among the Persians Mithras was the Light, and his worship was perhaps the purest cult that could be imagined. Later it was combined with sun worship, and Mithras became a Sun God, and as such generally recognized among the different peoples. To the early Greeks Mithras was unknown, but in the later days of the Roman Empire his mysteries made their appearance and gained great prominence. The monuments represented a young man in the act of slaying a bull with a dagger, while all around are human and animal figures, the youth standing for the Sun God who, on subduing Taurus in May, begins to develop his highest power. The original beautiful rites later degenerated and became orgies. Among the original rites was a form of baptism and the drinking of a potion made of meal and water. Human sacrifices were in some places a part of the cult.

The most disreputable of all these mysteries appear to have been the Sabazian, which were made up of several earlier forms, and were mere excuses for gluttony and lewdness, while the priests of the cult were most impudent beggars. Thus in time the mysteries were stripped of all the beauties of a heavenly origin and became of earth exceedingly earthy, while their initiates, lost to all shame and decency, persisted nevertheless in their sacred hypocrisy, until the hideous night of the Gods disappeared before the glow of a brighter morning. After this rather long preliminary portion, we are now prepared, as otherwise we could not be, to consider the relation between the Christian religion and these ancient mysteries. Granting that Jesus was the founder of the Christian religion, we must remember, nevertheless, that he was distinctly a Jew, spent his life in Judea, and based his teachings upon Judaism; also that long before his day Judaism was thoroughly indoctrinated with Greek elements, and that after his crucifixion the propaganda was carried on not so much by Jews as by Greeks and men of Grecian education. Between the Greeks and the Jews there were then, as now, the greatest differences; differences which have already been epitomized, but which may be thus summarized. On one side the closest union between God or the Gods and man, most lofty sentiments and finest sense of art-form, a priesthood making no pretentions and exerting little influence, a nation sustaining active commercial relations with the world, and all imbued with eagerness to adopt whatever was novel; on the other side, the widest separation between Jehovah and man, a substitution of theology and religious poetry for a study of nature, a nation ruled by priests and protected against all access from without, either by sea or caravan, adhering determinedly to the old and distrusting whatever was new.

After the Jews were liberated from Babylon, by Cyrus, they dispersed widely, living largely under Persian rule, and subjected after Alexander's conquest to Greek influences. Later they were scattered still more widely, becoming in time a mercantile race. In Egypt they enjoyed greater privileges than elsewhere, and in Alexandria saw the acme of Grecian art and teaching. While retaining their reverence for their scriptures and for the temple at Jerusalem, they quite generally adopted the language of the country, and particularly was this true of the Jews living in Alexandria in the third century, B. C, during which the Pentateuch was translated into the Septuagint, the remainder of the Hebrew bible being translated about 125 B. C. Thus the Greeks gained an introduction to Jewish theology, while the Hellenist Jews learned for the first time a Grecian philosophy; thus, too, among the scholars of one race was begotten a high esteem for the sages and philosophers of the other, while from the polytheism of one and the monotheism of the other was constructed a new mysticism. In this Alexandrian mysticism appeared in particular and for the first time the new idea of divine revelation, which was applied by enthusiasts alike to the Old Testament and to the Grecian writings. The Jew Aristobulus devised a most ingenious allegorical interpretation of the Old Testament, and traced to it all the wisdom of the Greeks, who until recently had never heard of it; and Philo, another Hebrew philosopher, contemporary with Christ, yet of whom he knew nothing, so construed the traditions of his race as to see in the four rivers of Eden the four cardinal virtues, in the trees of paradise the lesser virtues, and in the great figures of Jewish history personifications of various moral conceptions, all of which was out-doing the manner in which his Grecian friends had developed their own mysteries. Moreover, and this is very important, Philo taught that God had made a world of ideas and according to this model had subsequently made a corporeal world; the former having for its central point the Word. This statement that the Word was the first and the World his second deed passed later into the gospel of St. John, which opens "In the beginning was the word, and the word was God."

Philo founded a sect based upon the doctrine that the soul's union with the body is to be regarded as a punishment from which man should free himself, for his soul's sake. This sect was known as the Essenes, who in spite of claims to the highest antiquity really were founded during the first century B.C, and who constituted in effect a secret society. They were the true socialists of their day, and held things in common. They invented a peculiar nomenclature for the angels and imposed upon their new members to keep these names secret. As a society they did not long survive the beginning of the Christian era, being made superfluous by Christian asceticism. The Essenes, however, were of importance in this regard that they constituted the middle terms between the Grecian mysteries and Christianity, as they did between Grecian philosophy and Judaism. They were, in effect, a Jewish imitation of the Pythagorean league. When with Grecian mysticism were associated the nobility of Socrates, the philosophy of Plato, the science of Aristotle and the Jewish belief in one God, it is not strange that out of these elements, combined with the teachings of simple humanity enunciated by Christ, there resulted a power which transformed the world. The view that all mankind are brothers, originally Jewish, was also of independent Greek origin and came especially from the Stoics, who had to lie dormant until some tie stronger than mere political association held men together. This tie subsequently became a religious one. Polytheism had nothing more to give up; all the forces had been worked over in the God-making process, the Pantheon was full, and men ridiculed alike the Gods, their oracles and their priests. These same priests smiled at each other when they met, and forfeited all public respect by the lives they led. Olympic wantoning and derision of the Gods must necessarily have ended so soon as anything better could be substituted therefor.

The long felt want was for a God of definite character, of approved prowess, with human feelings, human wrath, and human love, made after man's own likeness, who should stand for a doctrine of personal immortality, and give some promise of a hereafter. The Jews, the only monotheists of the time, were prepared to furnish such a God, but he was too spiritual, and was worshiped by altogether too indefinite rites and peculiar usages. Nevertheless the God of the Jews was utilized for this purpose while the mystic elements with which he was to be surrounded were furnished by the ancient Grecian mysteries and the doctrines of the Pythagoreans and Essenes. So completely did the Jews and Greeks mingle in Egypt and In Judea, that the Idea prevailed among both races that the time had come for something new in the desired direction. The various secret leagues demanded a separation of the divine from the human and their subsequent reconciliation, all of which was subsequently furnished to their satisfaction in the accounts of the origin and death of Christ.. Even during the early years of the Roman Empire men looked for a new kingdom in the East, and both Jews and Heathen awaited some divine intervention. This took more definite form In the Jewish expectation of a Messiah who should restore the kingdom of Israel, and in their worship of Jehovah, while the Greeks yearned for something to take the place of their degenerate polytheism.

The times were thus ready for the appearance of Jesus, who lived for most of his life In obscurity, and of whose career no mention is made by contemporary Greek and Roman writers. This was perhaps fortunate for his followers, for none could contradict what any other might choose to say of Him who rose above the bigotry of his day and people, who was executed because of his independence of the priests and scribes, and who was thus regarded as the longed-for Messiah. On the Jewish branch of his real origin were grafted Grecian mystical offshoots of superhuman origin- an immaculate conception, a vicarious sacrifice, a resurrection and an assumption of a portion of the God-head. Thus, in what has come down to us concerning the Founder of the Christian church, truth and fiction mingle; the former being that which is consistent with highest laws and natural phenomena; and the latter that which conflicts with these. Jesus himself never made pretentions to being more than a man.

When he spoke of his father he spoke of him as equally the father of all mankind; he was the greatest moral reformer that ever lived, and he differed widely from the Essenes in that he sought to save man, not by Essenism and withdrawing him from the world, but by living with him and setting him a beautiful example. The ancients were firm believers In signs and portents from the heavens which were supposed to serve both for the instruction and warning of mankind. Stars, meteors, the aurora, comets and sudden lights of any kind were regarded as presaging events like the birth of Gods, heroes, etc. Great lights were supposed to have appeared both at the conception and birth of Buddha, and of Krishna. The sacred writings of China tell of like events In the history of the founder of her first dynasty, Yu, and of her inspired sages. The Greeks and Romans had similar traditions regarding the birth of Aesculapius and several of the Caesars. In Jewish history we read that a star appeared at the birth of Moses, and of Abraham- for whom an unusual one appeared in the East.

The prominence which a similar star in the East played in the legends of the Founder of Christianity and the effect which, as also in the case of Moses it had upon Magi, needs here no rehearsing. A very different significance was attached to eclipse or to any phenomena by which unexpected darkness is produced. The Greeks held that at the deaths of Prometheus, Hercules, Aesculapius and Alexander, a great darkness overspread the earth. In Roman history the earth was shadowed in darkness for six hours when Romulus died. Much the same thing is reported to have occurred when Julius Caesar died. So also one of the most conspicuous features attending the crucifixion of Jesus was a similar phenomenon which is made to play a most conspicuous part, for we read in three of the gospels that "darkness spread over the earth from the sixth to the ninth hour;" although the only evangelist who claims to have been present says nothing about it, nor do historians of that time, like Seneca and Pliny, make note of any such event in Judea.

In view of all this, however, to deny the star in the East, and the hours of darkness following the crucifixion, is regarded by many pious people as rank blasphemy or heresy of the deepest dye. The parables in which Jesus taught so unmistakably were similes adapted to the simple comprehension of his people, who likewise often made use of such figurative language. Those who followed him used this form of speech much more freely, and quickly erected his personality into the dignity of a God, magnified him and his mission, and soon saw him generally accepted as the equivalent of the Messiah, for whom Greeks and Jews alike had longed. His alleged miracles were unnecessary, in addition to being contradictory to all known natural sequences, because the simple and sublime truths which he preached could not be made more expressive by any such help. In the light of today they seem unnecessary juggleries, quite unworthy of so grand a character. They probably represent the effort of his followers, who portrayed his life and personality in colors which would make them more generally acceptable.

Of such transformations as that by which the son of a carpenter was made to appear of divine origin history has no lack. The Grecian polytheism furnished numerous illustrations; Apollo appeared on earth as a shepherd, Herakles, the son of Zeus, and Romulus (who was also the son of a virgin and of Mars), were founders of cities, states and nations. The Jewish accounts of creation stated that God walked the earth, and why not in human form? Why also should not the founder of a religion be the son of God and of a virgin? The rest of the beautiful story upon which we were all brought up must be regarded as fanciful embellishment, beautiful in its imagery, but having no foundation in fact or scientific possibility. The annunciation, the star in the East, the slaughter of the innocents, etc., can only be regarded in this light. The stories of the miracles are probably distinctively purposive. In the Grecian mysteries Demeter and Dionysos figured as givers of bread and wine; Jesus, too, was made lord and giver of these two sacred viands, all of which appears in his changing water into wine, multiplying the loaves, and later in the institution of the Last Supper, at which bread and wine became a part of these Christian mysteries which are still widely perpetuated. In his quieting the storm, walking upon the water, finding the penny in the fishes' mouth, and the draught of fishes, are portrayed his power over the forces of nature and lower forms of life. His power over disease was personified by stories of healing paralytics, lepers, blind, deaf and dumb people, casting out devils, and even by restoring the dead to life. Apparitions were common according to the history of his life, as of the holy spirit in form of a dove, his encounter with Satan, the appearance of Moses and Elias, etc. The ancient tendency to personify appears again in the form of Satan or a personal devil, namely the power of evil, while in the Transfiguration is personified the superiority of the new law over the old. Finally the miracles attending his last days, the darkening of the sun, the rending of the veil and the Resurrection, were all occurrences which it would be impossible to omit from the closing scenes in the life of anyone who has figured as a God. They betoken the mourning of nature, while the Ascension personified the belief in an everlasting Redeemer and the individual immortality of those who believed in him.

In thus epitomizing the events in the life of Jesus upon which, from his day until now, men have laid such fearful stress, and upon whose acceptance the present life as well as the future of all men has been conditioned, I should be far from doing justice to myself should I fail to point out my own attitude In the matter. I hold it true that the self-evident truth, as well as the wonderful sublimity of Christ's teachings, become apparent upon the study of the same, and are weakened rather than strengthened by insistence upon all that is supernatural, mysterious and inconceivable in the generally accepted account of his life and labor. My mind is freed from the necessity for the mysterious which the Greco-Jewish people demanded, and which the superstitious people of today still demand, and I prefer to let him stand for what he seems to me to be- the greatest moralist and teacher of all time, rather than to surround him with a veil of imagery and with statements so impossible of belief as to make it impossible to accept one part without accepting them all. The Jews already had doctrines of unity of God and love for others; the Grecian philosophy antedated him in insisting upon elevation of life to a higher plane than that of mere gratification of the senses, and everywhere his predecessors and contemporaries could furnish miracles by the hundred, but in force, grandeur and simplicity of his teachings, in his comprehensive humanity, in his directness of appeal, in his condemnations of those who departed from the model which he set, he never has had and probably never will have an equal. In his self-abasement and love for others he was as irresistible as have been these principles in civilizing and, in this sense, Christianize the world.

In Jesus' own day there was no hair-splitting theology; devotion, love of fellow-men, charity, repentance, these were all that were needed. But the beautiful simplicity of his teaching was lost with the death of his first disciples. The system was esteemed too simple, too unadorned to appeal to the people used to something quite the contrary. And so Stephen the Martyr, who was of Grecian education, was stoned because he demanded a repudiation of certain Jewish teachings, although the congregation at Antioch adopted his views. Paul the great leader was an epileptic and had frequent fits and visions, and these made a strong impression, not only on himself but on his followers. On the creations of his imagination the doctrine of the resurrection is largely based. He set up the Godman Jesus as the counterpart of the first man Adam, who represented sin and death, and who was to be crucified and born anew in Christ. Between Paul, the great Gentile Christian, and Peter, the Jewish Christian, the church was quickly split into two parties; these two soon subdividing into others, and among them all arose the New Testament literature, whose Alexandrine dialect establishes the influence of Greek education.

Thus did Christianity develop out of the secret associations of the ancient world. The early Christians themselves constituted, at least while under persecution, a sort of secret society. Their worship was mystical, but not because Jesus so taught- rather because of their environment and traditions. The practice of baptism, the last supper and the doctrines of incarnation and resurrection have been as certainly added to the Nazarene's sublime code of ethics as to them in turn, in the centuries to follow, were added every conceivable notion, mystery and stupid absurdity which the diseased minds of men could imagine, and which have been the cause of more departure from Christ's original teachings, and of more strife and bloodshed than any other feature in the history of mankind.

Indeed it is one of the greatest inconsistencies of history that the doctrines of love, unity and peace, taught by the Founder of Christianity, should have been the greatest of all factors to rend mankind apart, beget feelings of hatred, and result in the death, from this cause, of millions of men such as Jesus himself most loved.

THE EVIL EYE

VI: THE KNIGHTS HOSPITALLER OF ST. JOHN OF JERUSALEM

The three great militant, mendicant and monastic orders of the middle ages were the Knights Hospitaller of St. John, the Knights Templar, and the Teutonic Order. In addition were numerous others, smaller, shorter lived, less important in every respect, scarcely mentioned in even the larger histories, like the knights of Calatrava, Alcantara, Santiago de Compostella, and the English Knights of the Holy Sepulcher. These orders were the immediate as well as the indirect outgrowth of medieval conditions for which both the Church and the State were responsible. The secret tenets of the Christians had been made public, and those who held to them had for some time ceased to be a secret society; their faith was now a part of that church which was essentially the State, and which occupied a goodly part of Europe. Sad to say the Church was rent, and the State suffered accordingly from constant strife between sects and parties, who contested, even to the death, over interpretations to be given to the scriptures, and the matter of creeds. Thus while discussing at point of the sword whether the soul is to be saved by good works, or by grace of God, they disregarded the very essence of the simple teachings of Jesus, and brought upon theology, even in those days, the contempt and ridicule of the liberal minded and the non-believer, so that even today it suffers because of the unfortunate light in which it was made to appear. That theology should lead to war is the antithesis of the Christian doctrine, yet no wars have been so fierce and bloody as those waged in "spreading the cross" and propagating a misinterpreted gospel. And so theology suffered doubly from the Monks who perverted it, and from the Knights and the State that inculcated it with fire and sword.

For a thousand years nothing of importance was added to human knowledge, and mental confusion reigned supreme. At the end of this period all the original teachings of Christ were

93

forgotten, and after passing through the hands and tongues of fanatics or deluded and ignorant men, Christianity was left with the semblance of a monotheistic basis on which had been crudely built up certain doctrines borrowed from Egyptian and Grecian sources, among which may be mentioned the Trinity, Immaculate Conception, Resurrection and Ascension, as well as certain practices like that of the Lord's Supper, plainly borrowed from pagan customs. There was in all this so much to challenge belief, and so much at first unacceptable to minds not trained to believe it, that, in order to be effective their propaganda had to be carried on with the sword. Moreover to the Christian mystic, anxious to unify himself with the hidden, unknown deity, the idea of Moslem unbelievers in possession of the high places which they regarded with such reverence, was simply intolerable and repugnant beyond description.

Hence the Crusades undertaken in order to regain the Sepulcher; in which by Papal decree the Monks joined the Knights, and under command of emperors and the greatest generals of their day, made temporary conquest of the Holy Land, founding the kingdom of Jerusalem. The immediate outcome of the general movement was that alliance, made wise and even necessary, when theology and chivalry joined hands, from which resulted the foundation of such orders as those mentioned at the beginning of this paper. These allies of which they were composed, all took the monastic vows of poverty, chastity and obedience, and for a time kept them, until the possession of power and the acquisition of wealth brought their inevitably accompanying temptations. Each of these orders and many of the others passed through the successive stages of poverty, with meekness and constant benefaction, succeeded sooner or later by temporal aggrandizement, selfishness, greed, and rapacity, with all the crimes in the calendar, and the inevitable ultimate downfall. Of them all the Hospital Knights bore by all means the least smirched record, on which account, partly, as well as because of their most prominent purpose, i. e., their work among the sick, wounded and distressed, I deem their careers worthy of more particular study.

For this purpose we may quickly dismiss the Teutonic knights from present consideration, simply reminding you that they were really the founders of modern Prussia. They had their own origin in the commendable public spirit of the merchants of Lubeck and Bremen, who during the siege of Acre made tents out of the sails of their ships, in which their wounded countrymen might be nursed and attended. Most of their active service against the Saracens was in Spain. Of the Knights Templar a little must be said here. About 1119 two Knights, Hugo (or Hugh) of Payens, and Godfrey of St. Omers, associated with themselves six other French Knights in a league of military character, styling themselves "Poor Knights of Christ," and pledged themselves to keep safe for pilgrims the highways of the Holy Land. They prospered and grew, and came into the favor of Baldwin I, king of that kingdom of Jerusalem already mentioned. Inasmuch as their Monastery occupied a part of the site of Solomon's temple of old they were known as Templars. At the synod of Troyes, in 1128, they were recognized as a regular Order, and received monastic rules and habits, with a special banner.

They were also known as "Poor Companions of the Temple of Jerusalem," a name which did not very long befit them. At first, like the Hospital Knights, they begged their food, fasted, kept vows, worshiped diligently, and cared for the poor and infirm. Beard and hair were cropped short, the chase was forbidden, and they took the usual vows of chastity. But as they acquired property they forgot the simple life and habit, as well as their vows of obedience and chastity, while their pledge to protect the pilgrim on his way became in time a farce, not alone through their indifference and negligence, but through their treasonable dealings with the Saracens, and even treacherous surrender of their strongholds. Thus, whatever their pristine purpose, lucre and power became the later objects of their strife and the impelling motives of their lives. By the accession of so-called "affiliated members" they avoided the rule of celibacy, and admitted married knights and those engaged to be married.

Their Grand Masters in time ranked next after Popes and Monarchs. While the former favored them it was mainly because they feared them. They were exempt from all episcopal jurisdiction, and subject only to the Pope. So rich and powerful did they become that at the time of their suppression they controlled an Empire of five provinces in the East and sixteen in the West, while the Order possessed some 15,000 houses. They aimed to make' all Christendom dependent upon themselves, with only the Pope as their nominal head. Of their personal bravery, which was usually impeccable, of their affluence and intolerable effrontery, and of many of their traits and characteristics, one may form an excellent idea by reading Ivanhoe, where these seem to be quite faithfully depicted. It is, to me I confess, just a little amusing as well as saddening to see the men, who name their secret Masonic associations after the founders of the Order, displaying and imitating, at least in public where alone they can be judged by outsiders, only those features of Templar Knighthood which marked the period of their decadence or their downfall. As imitations they may be historically accurate, but as worthy of emulation, or even of imitation such displays are matters of questionable taste, at least, to those who read medieval history.

The Templars in their days of splendor and later downfall, were neither pious, nor learned, nor good Christians. Many of their secret doctrines were of heretical origin, taken from the Waldenses or the Albigenses, and they cared far more for their own possessions than for the Holy Land. They promulgated the shameful excuse that God evidently willed that the Saracen should win; that the defects of the Crusaders were evidently according to His decision, and that therefore they were released from their vows, and could return to Europe, where indeed they rested- after their fashion- from their labors, and passed their time in doing everything their founders had vowed not to do.

But this is not intended to be an epitome of Templar history; rather a brief statement of the reasons why they went proudly and sometimes stoically to their final downfall, and why the Hospital Order, though not always keeping up to its earlier standards, nevertheless so far eclipsed them, as to become the recipients of very much of the Templars' enormous resources and wealth, being thought worthy to be thus entrusted. And so it happened that, in 1307, Philip of France had all the Templars in France arrested and their property sequestrated. This led to a tripartite dispute in which were involved the Templars, the Pope and the King. In 1310 fifty-four Templar Knights were burned alive in Paris. At last the Pope, to prevent their property from falling into secular hands, made over to the Hospitallers most of the Templar estates, excepting however those in Spain. The Grand Master Molay and another Templar were burned to death on an island in the Seine. So much then in brief, for purposes of contrast. Now to the avowed subject of this paper.

During the seventeenth century there rose a controversy as to the foundation of a hospital already in existence in Jerusalem, named after the Asmorean prince John Hyrcanus, (the son and successor of Simon Maccabaeus, who restored the independence of Judea and founded a monarchy over which his descendants reigned till the accession of Herod. He died 105 B.C. This was at a time when the pious merchants of Amalfi planned a refuge for their pilgrims. It was this John whom many suppose to have been the patron of the order, though it seems now clearly established that the first sponsor or the first St. John, in this connection, was the Greek patriarch John surnamed Eleemon, or the Charitable, because of his practical philanthropy. (See "St. John the Almsgiver," Rev. H.T. F. Duckworth, 1901). But by the time the Crusaders, under Godfrey of Bouillon, had taken Jerusalem from the Saracens, St. John Baptist seems to have become the acknowledged patron saint of the hospital, his image being worn by epileptic patients, and being later adopted as the regular badge for those engaged in hospital work.

But this term hospital must not be regarded in its present acceptance; it was used in a broader sense to imply any house of refuge, even from wild animals; in fact a hospice. This particular hospice seems to have been erected on the ruins of one founded by St. Gregory in 603, where it is known that the French Benedictines worked. Two centuries later Charlemagne had claimed the title of Protector of the Pilgrims. ("De Prime Origine Hospitaliorum," by La Rouix. Paris. 1885). This institution was naturally located in close proximity to the most sacred places, which early Christian traditions made such to the pilgrims who came from all over Western Europe. It was in existence in 1099. It was made doubly necessary by not only the hardships of travel, but by the ill usage of the natives, at a time when the Holy City was in the hands of the Moslems, who demanded an entrance fee often beyond the pilgrims' means. Thus subjected to indignities indescribable, robbed often before their arrival, these misguided pilgrims often died of want, or returned with their primary pious object unattained. Had It not been for one Gerard, the first administrator of the hospice, their hardships had been even greater.

The buildings of the Order, at first meager, were finally enlarged to cover a square, nearly 500 ft. on each side, with one side on the Via Dolorosa and another fronting the Bazaar, and all a little south of the Church of the Holy Sepulcher. Nearby were other churches and hospices. This was the arrangement before the establishment of the kingdom of Jerusalem in 1099. During the next century the Order, under Raymond du Puy, had enlarged the church of St. John Eleemon Into the conventual church of St. John Baptist, while along the south of the square above mentioned ran an excellent building, the hospital of St. John. When Saladin recaptured Jerusalem, in 1187, this church was converted by the Turks Into a mad-house, known as the "Muristan," this being finally ceded to Germany In 1869.

THE EVIL EYE

From the new kingdom of Jerusalem the Hospitallers obtained a constitution, and the Gerard above mentioned was made their first "Master." He was succeeded In 1118 by du Puy, while Baldwin II was the Latin King of Jerusalem. The Hospital had been recognized by the Archbishop of Caesarca in 1112, and had widely extended Its sphere of uscfulness. It was King Baldwin who was anxious to stamp upon the Order a military character, similar to that conferred upon the Order of the Temple In 1130. This was natural since the kingdom was isolated, surrounded by fanatic enemies and always beset by and in danger from them. Thus the necessities of the times and the environment made it requisite that all who were able should bear arms, and cooperate for mutual defense.

Thus it came about that the Order was divided into three divisions, the first in rank being the lights of Justice, each of whom must be of noble ink or birth, and have received the accolade of knighthood from secular authority. The second division comprised the ecclesiastics, who were later divided into two grades, the Conventual Chaplains, who were assigned to duty at headquarters, and the Priests of Obedience who served other priories and commanderies in various parts of Europe. The third grade were the Serving Brothers, also divided into the Servants at arms or Esquires, and the Servants at office. The Servants at arms attended the Knights of Justice as their Esquires, and might eventually become eligible to the first division. The Servants at office were little if anything more than menials or domestics. Even these latter, however, possessed certain privileges and emoluments which made admission to this grade advantageous to men of humble origin and faculties.

The dress of the Order was a black robe with cowl, having a white linen cross of eight points over the left breast, and was at first worn by all. Later, under Pope Alexander IV, the fighting knights wore their white crosses upon a ground gules. The first recorded appearance of a body of Hospitaller knights in actual war was at Antioch, in 1119, while the complete military constitution of the Order of St. John was achieved in 1128. During the balance of the existence of the Kingdom of Jerusalem then, two colleges or companies of military monastic knights existed, side by side, in the Holy Land, the "chief props of a tottering throne." (Bedford).

Between these rival bodies arose in time such jealousy, and within them such intrigues- aggravated always by the animosities of the ordinary clergy, who took offense at the patronage bestowed upon the orders by the Popes, aggravated also by similar difficulties on the part of the knights of the Teutonic Order and that of St. Lazarus- that the best interests of the kingdom and of the Church suffered as much from intestine dangers as from those arising from the Moslems surrounding them. Nevertheless it may be said that the Order of the Hospital never lost sight of its primary purposes, and never disgraced itself by the treasonable and treacherous dealings, and correspondence with enemies which disgraced not a few members of other and rival Christian organizations. The result of such disreputable actions lead- as ever- to disunion and final disruption, and this to final capitulation and surrender of Jerusalem, in 1187. This meant the abandonment not only of their old home, but of their usefulness there. The Saracens occupied their buildings and premises from that time till ruin overtook them. Thus rudely compelled to emigrate the Order moved the same year (1187) to the town of Margat, where was also a castle of the same name. But the work in Jerusalem had not been abruptly discontinued, since Sultan Saladin, In evidence of his esteem, allowed them possession of their hospital for another year, in order that their charitable work should not be abruptly Interrupted, and even made them liberal donations. When during the third Crusade, In which Richard Coeur de Lion bore so valiant a part, Ptolemais was captured. It was then and there that the Order established its headquarters, In 1192, wherefore the town became named St. Jean d'Acre. Here they abode nearly a century.

THE EVIL EYE

Various other towns In Palestine held out for a time against the Turks, e. g., Carac, Margat, Castel Blanco and Antioch, and in spite of the intense rivalry between the Orders, Thierry, the Grand Master of the Templars, reported in a letter to King Henry II, that the Hospitallers bore themselves even with fervor and the greatest bravery, and praised the aid they gave in the capture of the Turkish fleet, at Tyre, when seventeen Christian galleys manned by friars, and ten Sicilian vessels commanded by General Margarit, a Catalan, defeated the Infidels, and captured their admiral and eight Emirs, with eleven ships, the rest being run aground, where Saladin later burned them, to keep them from falling Into Christian hands. (Bedford).

Notwithstanding all this, however, the joint occupation of Acre with the Templars had a bad effect on both Orders, who turned not only to luxury and license, but their swords against each other. Acre was at this time a most cosmopolitan city; here mingled at least seventeen different nationalities and languages, each occupying its own part of the city, so that in time extravagance and lust flourished to the last degree of demoralization. The Hospitallers were at this time far more wealthy than the Templars, who were exceedingly jealous thereof, and both at Margat and still worse at Acre this jealousy was exhibited in many bloody affairs. Weakened thus by this intestine strife they were in reverse proportion strengthened. The Pope who had defended them as against the scathing censure of Emperor Frederick, found need, in 1238, to accuse the knights-alike of both orders- of sheltering loose women within their precincts, of owning individual property, both of these in violation of their vows of chastity and poverty, and of treacherously assisting the enemy. Yet many bore witness to the actual good they accomplished, even at this time. In 1259 Pope Alexander, bewailing the lack of a more distinctive dress, permitted the decree that the fighting knights might wear black mantles, while in war they were permitted to wear red surcoats, with a white cross.

THE EVIL EYE

Later it was permitted to women to join the Order, and many ladies of high degree took advantage of the permission, rivaling in religious zeal and in charitable deeds the most sanctified of the brethren. As the King of Hungary wrote, at one time, after visiting some of their houses, "In a word the Knights of St. John are employed, sometimes like Mary in contemplation, and sometimes like Martha in action, and this noble militia consecrate their days either in their infirmaries or else in engagements against the enemies of the cross."

The deterioration of Acre was not so great as to make cowards of our Knights, however, and with the continued and aggressive siege laid by the Saracens against that city the Hospitallers and the Templars finally made common cause, each endeavoring to outdo the other in deeds of bravery and daring. Though defeated again and again, the Moslem ranks were renewed by fresh soldiers, while the militant and other monks imprisoned within the city saw their combined members steadily diminish. At last it remained for John Villiers, Grand Master, with his few surviving fighters, to carve their way to their boats, leaving no combatants behind them, and then to embark in their galleys to seek a harbor of refuge in the island of Cyprus. Cyprus and Rhodes. Settled in Cyprus, the Knights renewed their zeal and their resources. Here they began to build that fleet of galleys which, increased later in Rhodes, became most formidable. When they and the Templars left forever the Holy Land the Templars took the position that their vow to protect the holy places was now either fulfilled or at least at an end, and they distributed themselves among their numerous preceptories all over Europe, where they made themselves *personae non gratae* to their civil rulers, because of their own real power, their oriental ostentation, and their secularization and distasteful entrance into and interference with the social and political life and customs of their new environment.

Things went from bad to worse, public feeling was more and more aroused, and their extermination was only a matter of time. Finally Pope Clement V and King Phillip le Bel undertook this task with barbarous ruthlessness. Kings, nobility and the people joined hands in the common task. The Templars had acquired various properties, by capture, by bequest, and in every lawful and unlawful manner, which yielded in the aggregate relatively enormous revenues, too strong a temptation for needy secular rulers to resist. The Pope had at last to intervene in order to prevent the total secularization of all this great spoil, and thus it happened that no small proportion of it was, after its sequestration, allotted to the Order of St. John, whose Grand Masters and Knights had not forgotten nor abandoned their original vows and purposes, and who held that the inviolacy of their obligations required their continuous residence in some such oriental city as Rhodes.

And here we may part company, as did they, only quite peacefully, with the Templar Knights. Driven from Europe they made their last stand in Great Britain, and of their lives and deeds there we have no more readable nor interesting historical account than Scott has given us in Ivanhoe. Any further allusion to them here will be most casual. They offer the conventional picture, only *in extenso*, of original poverty and self-abnegation, coupled with devotion and valor, changed to arrogance, treason, abandonment of purpose, unbridled lawlessness leading to crime and cruelty, all brought about because of affluence, acquired power, selfishness, cupidity and every debasing human weakness. Small wonder then, that they could be no longer tolerated in Christendom. So turn we again to the Hospitallers, now made rich and powerful at the expense of their old rivals and at last enemies. It had soon been made evident that Cyprus did not meet their wants and necessities. Its king was not over friendly, and they sought further.

Their gaze fixed on the island of Rhodes, which possessed a fertile soil, a city with an excellent harbor, not too far from the main land, i. e. not too isolated, which was under the- by that time merely nominal- suzerainty of the Emperor of the Eastern or Greek empire. After several futile efforts they at last, in 1310, under the twenty-fourth Grand Master Villaret, captured the island, where under their ceaseless energy both hospitals and forts were built. To Rhodes were brought also Christian refugees from the various Turkish provinces, and thus their numbers were rapidly strengthened. Their fleet, already begun (*vide supra*) was greatly increased, and with it they had many a conflict with the Turkish corsairs, whose inroads they practically checked.

About the beginning of the fourteenth century changes had been made in the Order, which was now divided into Langues, or arranged according to nationalities, yet without materially altering the original division into the three classes (Knights, Chaplains and Serving Brothers). In this way the Order was apportioned between seven nations or languages, Provence, Auvergne, France, Italy, Aragon, England and Germany. Finally under pressure from Spain the Langue of Aragon was divided into two, Aragon and Castile, the latter including Portugal. The various dignities and offices were divided among these langues, whose principals became a kind of Privy Council to the Grand Master, and were known as Conventual Bailiffs. They were given different names in each country; thus the Grand Commander of the English langue was known as the Turcopolier, of France the Grand Hospitaller, of Italy the Admiral, etc. As the new fortifications arose around the city of Rhodes, each was placed in charge of one of these langues or divisions, while each erected quarters for its own men. It did not follow, however, that every member of each langue came from the country which it represented. While Scotland was an independent kingdom it contributed to the Turcopolier, while many Scotchmen belonged to the French or even the other langues. At this time the inhabitants of the City of Rhodes consisted largely of Christian refugees, who owed their security, even their lives, to the fact that the Knights Hospitaller still adhered to their primary objects, the liberation of the captive and giving assistance to the sick and distressed. This they afforded through their fleet and their hospices. When Smyrna nearly fell into the hands of Timour the Tartar, about the middle of the fourteenth century, the Order strengthened their harbor by erecting a new fort, which they named Budrum (corrupted from Petros-a Rock), where any Christian escaping from slavery found shelter. Here was also kept a remarkable breed of dogs, who were trained not only as watch dogs but to render services similar to those afforded by the Alpine dogs of St. Bernard.

As time went on the Sultans became more and more jealous of the naval power possessed by the Order. With the fall of the Eastern Empire and the final retaking of Constantinople by Mahomet II, in 1453 (See "Prince of India"), it was made evident that danger to the Order from this direction was rapidly increasing. This became so urgent that in 1470, after Mahomet had taken the island of Negropont, the Grand Master commanded that all members of the Order should repair at once to Rhodes. In 1476 d'Aubusson began the most active measures for the defense of the place, and thus was ready for the attack, in May, 1480, when 80,000 men in 160 ships, landed on the island coast. In this siege no small part was played by renegade traitors, the most prominent being one George Frapant, a German, whom the Grand Master finally hung in July. In the last sorties which terminated this siege deeds of the greatest bravery were performed; yet here we can only commemorate the fact that the Turks were summarily defeated, leaving 3,500 corpses on the ground after the last decisive attack. The losses of the besieged were small as compared with those suffered by the Turks.

Later in the same year the island suffered from a severe earthquake. Mahomet died not long after this, was succeeded by his son Bo-jazet who made truce with the Order, presenting them with a relic of supposedly inestimable value, namely the hand of St. John, which the Turks had taken at Constantinople. Years of comparative quietude succeeded until in the following century, in 1522, Solyman the Magnificent landed upon the island in July, with 100,000 soldiers and 60,000 pioneers. Again ensued all the horrors of a siege. The defenders did their part so bravely that the Sultan publicly disgraced his generals. But the inevitable famine wrought consequent disaffection on the part of the native population, who clamored for capitulation, and sought treasonable terms therefor, because of which one of the most prominent of them was tried, found guilty and executed. Finally under stress of circumstances no longer endurable Grand Master Adam agreed to honorable surrender, and on the first of January, 1523, the Hospitaller Knights relinquished the island, the Sultan himself speaking in terms of extravagant praise of their heroism, while at the same time he scathingly censured the Christian monarchs of Europe who had failed to come to their relief. Thus after two hundred and twenty years of occupation and rule of the Island of Rhodes, some 5,000 Knights and other members of the Order, and natives, left it to take abode for a short time in their Pridry at Messina. Driven from here by plague, they moved on to Viterbo, while their Grand Master traveled in search of a new home.

Malta: Malta had been early proposed for this purpose, and offered by Charles V, while many wishes turned to the city of Modon, in Greece. After seven years of wandering and indecision Grand Master L'Isle Adam accepted Malta as the best solution of the difficulty. Thither the Order now removed, and there Adam died in the Castle of St. Angelo, erected by the Norman Count Roger of Sicily, still active in improving its existing defenses. In 1555 the Order lost nearly all of its fleet in consequence of a violent hurricane, which accident for a while laid the island open to piratical attacks, especially of a corsair named Dragut; but he did little damage, save that with the knowledge of the island and its defenses thus gained he persuaded Solyman to undertake another attempt to crush the Order, the latter being justly furious because some galleys belonging to the Order had captured a ship that happened to be loaded with rich valuables belonging to the ladies of his harem. Therefore war was again declared in 1565.

THE EVIL EYE

The Turkish fleet was made up of 130 galleys with 50 smaller boats, and carried the Janissaries and 34,000 other soldiers, against whom the Grand Master could only oppose some 9,000 men,700 of whom, however, were desperate men, released from the galleys of the enemy, and eager for vengeance. On May twenty-fourth the siege of St. Elmo was in reality begun by a fierce bombardment, the walls being soon battered, and the garrison forced to take shelter in excavations made in the solid rock. And now the besiegers' force was augmented by the arrival of Dragut, in those days the dreaded corsair of the sea, who came with thirteen more ships and 1,500 more men. June thirteenth saw a desperate conflict when, after six hours of fierce fighting and the loss of only 300 men, the besiegers were repulsed. Soon after this Dragut was killed. Again on June twenty-third another general attack was repulsed, though the garrison was thereby reduced to 60 men. Even this small force, many crippled and maimed, repulsed the first onslaught of the Turks, but had later to sell their lives as dearly as they could.

The Turkish general Mustapha took barbarous revenge, even on the corpses of the Knights which he decapitated and then tied to planks that they might float past St. Angelo. La Vallette retaliated by beheading some of his captives and firing their heads at the Turks from his cannon. At this juncture the garrison was reinforced by the arrival of 700 men and 42 Knights from Sicily. Refusing all opportunities to surrender and all parley under flags of truce. Grand Master La Vallette built new defenses and strengthened the old, in spite of a fierce July sun. Meanwhile the Turks, also reinforced, prepared for still more desperate sorties, selecting for the land attack men who knew not how to swim, in order that they might fight the more fiercely, and drawing off the boats as soon as their loads were emptied, so that no retreat could be possible. One thousand Janissaries were embarked in ten large barges, but nine of these were sunk by the artillery fire from the forts. On the other side of the defenses a large attacking column was completely routed. The . loss to the Turks this day was 3,000 men, that of the garrison 250.

And so the siege went on; attack after attack, with but small success to the investing army. But the heroic defenders suffered increasingly under the constant strain, and both armies were exhausted, the Turks losing 800 men from dysentery alone. To such an extent was this true that when the Turkish officers drove their soldiers to the charge by blows of their own swords, it was but necessary to cut down those who led the charges, when the rest would turn and fly. And now came other long expected reinforcements from Sicily, when a fleet landed 8,500 men and returned for 4,000 more. Being now quite unequal to the continuation of the siege the Turks evacuated all the ground they had gained, and finally made a hasty and complete flight, harassed in every way, in their endeavors to escape, by the now victorious garrison. The losses during the period of siege, with its numerous engagements, were estimated at some 30,000 Turks, and 8,000 men and 260 Knights of the Order.

Is it strange that by contributions from all over Christian Europe there was soon built up a town bearing the name of Valetta, thus commemorating the heroism and military prowess of the Order's Grand Master La Valette, as well as the "glorious issue" of the struggle for Malta, and the confirmation of the Order as a sovereign independent community?

Thus secured from further probable struggle this city of Valetta acquired a certain degree of glory, later even of magnificence. From all parts of Europe, wherever any commandery of the Order was maintained, was paid tribute to the Grand Master, as may be adjudged even today, long after French rapacity had robbed the city of many of its treasures. Individual Knights vied with each other in their gifts, and palaces arose wherein were received the envoys and even ambassadors of foreign courts. The fleet was constantly busied in clearing the Mediterranean of Moslem and other pirates, and many Christians were released from the galleys in which they had been chained to the oars. In this restoration the English langue took a rather small part, and their officers and members had often to be rebuked or punished for insubordination or worse crimes. The Reformation In England Interfered, and furnished some reason for their diminishing zeal. The galleys of the Order became more and more like pleasure boats, and many of their cruises were in effect pleasure excursions. Later in their decadence their adventures became more like piratical incursions, until, under letters of marque issued by a decadent Admiralty, the Malta privateer was equivalent to the pirate. (Maroyat). These facts were scarcely offset by that other, that the last fleet of the Order, which left Valetta in 1783, was sent to the relief of earthquake sufferers in Sicily.

With regard to their activities in the matter of succoring the sick let it be noted that the Knights found on their arrival at Malta a hospital or hospice already existing. In the buildings of a nunnery still standing may be seen the gateway of their own first hospital. In 1575 they erected one much larger, which had a passageway connected with the waterfront, so that patients could be brought directly from the ships. This building in some part still remains in use as a military hospital. Its great ward is 500 feet in length, and 30 feet high, divided by partitions 15 feet in height. In its best days patients were served from silver utensils. It was under the charge of the Regent of the French Knights, who had as his staff five doctors and three apothecaries. Other knights and servants acted as male nurses. The knights were luxuriously cared for, and 150 beds were always in reserve for those returning from expeditions who might need them.

In 1796, only a year before the disintegration of the Order began, the patients numbered from 350 to 400. There existed also a hospital for women, with 230 beds, and a foundling hospital where some fifty waifs were sheltered. A curious bit of history connecting the middle ages with the more recent past relates to the hospital interests of the Order. The nobles of Dauphigny had founded a fraternity of Hospitallers for the relief of sufferers from St. Anthony's fire (erysipelas), which was erected into the regular Antonine order in 1218. About 550 years later, or to be exact in 1777, a compact was made by which the Order of St. John took over their property, under certain conditions, which involved, among other considerations, a larger expenditure. The Antonine estates, in France and Savoy, were confiscated In 1792, thus entailing a tremendous loss to the Order, so great, in fact, that the Valetta treasury became insolvent. (Bedford). From this time we may date the rapid downfall of the Order. Malcontents and traitors gained the supremacy, and in 1798, after treacherous negotiations. Napoleon landed part of his army in Malta, and Valetta surrendered.

Thus, as Bartlett says, "ignominiously came to a close, on June 12th, 1798, the once illustrious Order of St. John of Jerusalem, having subsisted for more than 700 years."

At this time it consisted of 328 enrolled knights, and a military force of some 7,000 men. Napoleon expressed his surprise at the strength of the fortifications, furnished them with one thousand cannon, left a garrison of 3,000 men, took with him the disciplined soldiers he found there, rifled the island of its treasures, its art work and its bullion, and sailed for Egypt. Several of the traitor knights were put to death by the infuriated populace, whose anger was not appeased by Nelson's victory at Aboukir- the battle of the Nile- but took form in open insurrection. The French garrison finally took refuge in the old fortifications, where they withstood for two years a siege by the combined insurgents and an English fleet. Finally reduced by famine and disease they capitulated to the English forces under Gen. Pigot. The latter then selected Capt. Sir Alexander Ball, Nelson's representative. Governor of the Island. At the Peace of Amiens the effort was made to restore the Order as ruling authority, under the protectorate of the Great Powers, but the Maltese themselves objected so vehemently that after no small amount of trouble and dispute the Inhabitants of the island elected to place themselves under the sovereignty of Great Britain, an arrangement finally and definitely confirmed at the Congress of Vienna In 1814.

Thus disappeared from history one of the most interesting and longest enduring institutions recorded in its pages, and certainly the most long-lived of any of its kind. I say disappeared, meaning thereby only to indicate its disruption, as it were into fragments, its primary purpose, i.e. aid to the needy, being kept ever in view by some, while others preferring the life of a soldier, took service under various rulers or military leaders. The traitors who were responsible for surrender to Napoleon fared badly according to their deserts, though it does not appear that any of them were hung. In the migration England seemed to attract many, perhaps the majority of those who were still inclined to good deeds. The title of Grand Master was still continued, under some pretension to perpetuation of the Order. In Russia the Czar Alexander, in 1801, upon the death of his predecessor Paul, announced himself a Protector of the Order, and designated Count Soltikoff to exercise the functions of the Grand Master.

Thus dismembered, disunited and scattered, the fragmentary langues of the Order underwent, on their way to final dissolution, various vicissitudes, through which they cannot here be followed. Complete extinguishment was the eventual fate of most of them. I shall only concern myself now with that of the English langue, and its partial revival in 1830. Rev. Dr. Peat, chaplain to George IV, was one of those to whom the remnants of the English langue appealed, with the result that in 1827 certain notable English gentry, of eminent attainments, undertook to revive the Order in England, only under quite different conditions from those previously obtaining. In 1831 Dr. Peat was invested with the authority and functions of Grand Prior. It will be at once seen how the matter of religious belief now separated the English Order from all the survivors of the previous regime, and why the last ties were severed. Under the new regime members of the Order dropped all pretense of playing a military role; one may read thereafter of real hospital activity. The Life Boat movement and ambulance work were gradually incorporated into their plans and scope. When First Aid to the Injured began to be publicly taught public and general interest was quickly aroused, and the energetic cooperation of eminent men was assured. In other words the Order gradually took up just that class of work which is now done under the Red Cross.

Sir Edward Lechmere established, in 1867, a commandery of the Order in one of his castles, and in 1874 was instrumental in the acquisition of the St. John Gate, which still stands, an example of Tudor architecture as also a well preserved monumental relic of the time, beginning about 1180, when the Order had founded a hospital in Clerkenwell, while the ladles of the order were housed in Bucland, in Somersetshire. The old Priory of the Order in Clerkenwell was practically destroyed In 1381, by the mob led by Jack Straw, in an insurrection which had, along with other results, as an incident, the beheading of Sir Robert Hales, the Prior of the Order. In the slow process of rebuilding the present Gate was not completed till 1504. On the North and South fronts remain projecting towers, while in the Western tower a spiral stair case is still in use. Bedford's work, from which I have drawn heavily, gives excellent pictures of the Gate as it appears today, and of the old priory restored.

Colonel Duncan, also, deserves honorable mention in this connection; he became Director of the Ambulance Movement In 1875. Finally we have to record here that under a new Charter, granted in 1888, the then Prince of Wales, later King Edward, became the Grand Prior. Therefore the Order of the Hospital, in England of St. John of Jerusalem is, in fact, the legitimate successor- one might say the lineal descendant- of the old Order of Knights Hospitaller, though It is today a secular and voluntary society, keeping to the traditions of the past, no longer military nor militant, save as it fights disease and best of all teaches others how to do the same. To follow it further is no longer necessary. Its work is essentially that of the Red Cross. It has, for instance, a depot at old St. John's Gate, whence all the material required in teaching and illustrating as well as rendering first aid is issued. Its work was begun with a two-wheeled litter, an old Esmarch triangular bandage from Germany, and a stretcher from France. Now It distributes all these things throughout the British Empire. Now, too, it maintains ambulances all over the city of London, which do for their own hospitals just what each of our hospitals at home has to do for itself. The German "Samariter-Verein" is virtually a Chapter of the English Order in its revivified form. In 1883 a branch of the Order was organized in India, where among others the native police are instructed in "First Aid." In 1882, by a Fireman of the Turkish Sultan, an Ophthalmic Hospital was opened, under the auspices of the Order, in Jerusalem. Only those who have traveled in the East can appreciate what this means to the poor, where squalor vies with ignorance, and, as in Egypt though not so universally, both conspire to the ruin of that greatest of all blessings- eyesight.

But I will not delay to write further of what the Ambulance Brigade of London, and its affiliated corps, have accomplished in many parts of the world; in South Africa, for example, it works under the general supervision of the Order of St. John, as it now exists in London. It does everything that in our country is accomplished by the Red Cross for the general public, and by the Hospital Corps and their Medical Officers for our Army and Navy. Over the graves of eleven members of the brigade, who died at their posts in South Africa, in St. Paul's, London, not far from the crypts where lie the remains of Nelson and Wellington, has been erected a monument to their; memory. Another bearing among other inscriptions this beautiful scriptural quotation: "Greater love hath no man than this, that he lay down his life for his friends," was unveiled by His Royal Highness, acting as Grand Prior, in St. John's Church, Clerkenwell, June 11th, 1902. Fifteen hundred men enrolled in the Order had left that church before their departure for the Front, and of these about seventy sacrificed their lives to this sort of duty. Do not the dead deserve all praise and respect, and the survivors all commendation?

A few years ago my friend Sir George Beatson, surgeon to the Royal Infirmary in Glasgow, published a little monograph-"The Knights Hospitallers in Scotland and their Priory at Torphichen" (Printed by Hedderwick and Sons, Glasgow,)-which aroused my interest sufficiently to prompt a visit to this, the last home of the old Order in that part of the world. The little village Torphichen lies about midway between Glasgow and Edinburgh, and three miles south from the town of Lunlithgow. Here had been founded, in 1124, one of the great Priories or Preceptories under control of the English langue. Here they settled in a magnificent and fertile area, the Grampian hills to their north; to their west could be seen the snow-capped top of what is now known as Ben Lomond. By donation, by cultivation of the arable soil, and by wise management of their resources, they prospered greatly, from the worldly point of view.

Here they erected that building, a part of which still exists, and which makes a picturesque ruin which is not yet a scene of desolation. The members of the Order took, here as elsewhere, the view that the best way to serve God was by remaining in it and working, not by fleeing from it into lazy, selfish and profitless solitude as did too many of the monks. In common with other monasteries the Torphichen Preceptory possessed the Right of Sanctuary, and in its churchyard still stands the short stone pillar, carved with a Maltese cross on its upper surface, which meant that within a mile in every direction therefrom all those charged with any crime, save murder only, might find temporary protection. Here for four hundred years, and until the Reformation upset everything, the Hospitallers carried on their affairs. In 1560 their last Preceptor or Grand Prior made over to the Crown all their properties and effects. The Crown in return made these possessions a temporal Barony, carrying with it the title of Lord of Torphichen. From this time the property began to suffer- from time, storm, vandalism of the people and neglect. Still the present Lord Torphichen has proven himself a better guardian than did some of his predecessors. A parish church has been built, partly upon the sight of the old structure, partly into it. Dr. Beatson has urged that a combination between the present Order of St. John, in London, and the St. Andrew's Ambulance Association might be effected which might work to the benefit of both, by reviving some of the work done here in days gone by. I have ventured this brief reference to Torphichen, partly because of my interest in the place itself, associated with my visit there, and partly because every such visit to the monuments of past grandeur and usefulness should strengthen our interest and zeal in what man is accomplishing today, and should help link together the Past and the Present in a manner not merely fascinating but inspirational, and keep us from forgetting that motto of the Order.

Pro utilitate Hominum

For the Welfare of Mankind

THE EVIL EYE

VII: GIORDANO BRUNO

The renaissance was the fourth of the great events in the history of the Christian Era; the first being the decline of Rome, the second the introduction of the Christian cult, and the third, the intrusion into Southern Europe of the Teutonic and Slavonic tribes. With none of these however, save the fourth, is this paper primarily concerned, and not even with the fourth save indirectly, though it deals with a special feature of it. Protestants and Catholics alike impeded progress and the self-evolution of reason in every possible way. Italy gave the world the Roman Republic, then the Roman Empire and finally the Roman Church; after that arose a new storm center in the North which swept toward the Mediterranean. The Teutons effaced the Western Empire, adopted Christianity, and completely modified what remained of Latin civilization. Then the Roman Bishops separated the Latin from the Greek Church, and under the captious title of The Holy Roman Empire bound Western Europe into what has been called a "cohesive whole."

While Romans and Teutons never actually blended homogeneously, they had yet a common bond of union. When this coalition was for a time freed from both Papacy and Empire-then began intellectual activity and Independence of thought, taking form in Italy as the Renaissance; in Germany as the Reformation. In the South it was known as the Revival of Learning. It furnished a *lux a non lucendo*, Italy gave freedom rather to the mind, Germany rather to the soul. Toward the South men still took refuge behind that form of modified paganism which became Catholicism. In the North they attained a more complete emancipation because of their violent opposition to the Papacy and all that went with it. In the long run both attained the same result, i. e., liberation of the mind from artificial impediments and fetters, though they of the North achieved it in its full extent far earlier. (I am speaking of course, relatively; men's minds are far from free even today, but the state we have reached Is a great advance upon that of Bruno's time). The Reformation led men to be far more outspoken than they dared be in the South; the free thinkers of Italy were still content to do homage to a thoroughly corrupt Papal hierarchy. As critics and warriors Luther and Calvin rank as liberators of the human mind, but later, as founders of mutually hostile sects, they only retarded civilization, and the churches they founded are today as stagnant pools. In 1548, in the midst of this stormy period in Italian history Bruno was born, In the little village of Nola, not far from Naples, whence Vesuvius was visible In the picturesque distance. His father was a soldier, his mother of very humble origin. Of his family history nothing Is known ; little explanation is thus afforded, by the doctrine of heredity, for the marvelous mental faculties which he subsequently displayed.

Nevertheless his father was a man of some culture, at least, for he was a friend of Tansillo, a poet, under whose Influence the growing boy subsequently came. Bruno has told us himself how one Savolino (probably an uncle) annually confessed his sins to his Cure, of which "though many and great" his boon companion readily absolved him. But only once was full confession necessary; each subsequent year Savolino would say: "Padre mio, the sins of a year- today- you may know them;" to which the Cure would reply "son, thou knowest the absolution of one year ago- go In peace, and sin no more."

In those days as in many others superstition was everywhere rife and effective. Its influence must not be disregarded as one studies the formation of Bruno's character. When he was about eleven years old Bruno was sent to Naples to be taught logic, dialectics and humanities. When fifteen he entered the Dominican Monastery in Naples, and assumed the clerical habit of that order. Here he gave up his baptismal name of Filippo and assumed that of Giordano, according to the monastic custom. In 1572 he was ordained priest. His reasons for thus entering the Church are scarcely far to seek. Of Intellectual bent, and studious rather than martial in his habits and inclinations, there was but one career open to him. To be sure the Dominican Order was the most narrow and most bigoted of all, as the current punning expression "Domines" will indicate. Still it was at that time the most powerful, especially in the kingdom of Naples, which was then ruled by Spain. The old cloister had been once the home of St. Thomas Aquinas, whose works Bruno claimed at his trial he had always by him, "continually reading, studying and restudying them, and holding them dear."

This was the age when efforts to put down every heresy had been redoubled. The fanaticism of Loyola, and the decision of the Council of Trent "to erase with fire and sword the slightest traces of heresy," made a poor frame work in which to place the picture of a liberal minded scholar. Bruno soon learned this at his cost. Even during his novitiate he was accused of giving away images of the saints, and of giving bad advice to his associates. In 1576 he was accused of apologizing for the heresy of Arlus, that the Son was begotten of the Father, and so not consubstantlal nor coeternal with Him, but created by Him and subordinate to Him; (which was condemned by the Council of Nice, 325, and contradicted in the Nicene Creed;) admiring its scholastic form, rather than its abstract truth. Disgusted with his treatment he left Naples and went to Rome. Even here he was molested In the Cloister of Minerva (note the pagan name), and was met with an accusation of 130 specifications. He then abandoned his garb and his cloister and escaped from Rome, beginning thus the nomadic life which he continued until immured in the dungeons of the Inquisition at Venice, sixteen years later. Through these wanderings one must follow him, if one would become familiar with his life and traits.

He now resumed for a time his baptismal name, and traveled to a town on the Gulf of Genoa, where he taught youth and young gentlemen. Then he passed on to Turin and Venice, where he spent weeks in futile attempts to find work. But the schools and the printing houses were closed because of the plague. In Venice however he managed to print his first book on

"The Signs of the Times;" or rather this was his first book to appear in print. It seems that before he left Naples he wrote "The Ark of Noah," a satirical allegory. In this he represented that the animals held a formal meeting in the Ark, to settle questions of precedence and rank, and that the presiding officer, the Ass, was in danger of losing his position and his influence, because his power lay rather in hoofs than horns. Throughout most of his life Bruno constantly scored and criticized Asinity; it was frequently the topic of his invective, and those who read between his lines were probably quite justified in regarding these frequent allusions as references to the ignorance, bigotry and credulity of the Monks.

From Venice Bruno went to Padua, where some of the Dominican friars persuaded him to resume monastic costume, since it made travel easier and safer. Thence by way of Brescia and Milan he may be followed to Bergamo. At Milan he first heard of his future friend Sir Philip Sydney. From Bergamo he resolved to go to Lyons, but learning that he would find anything but welcome there he turned aside and crossed the Alps, arriving in Geneva in the Spring of 1579. Here he was visited by a distinguished Neapolitan exile, the Marquis De Vico, who persuaded him again to lay aside his clerical garb, and who gave him the dress of a gentleman, including a sword. Here is raised the great question- Did Bruno adopt Calvinism? Before the Inquisition fifteen years later he practically denied this, yet acknowledged attending the lectures of Balbani, of Lucca, as well as of others who taught and preached in Geneva. Under the regulations of the Academy (University), where he had already registered, certain regulations must be complied with, and Bruno appears to have obeyed them in at least a certain degree. But the immediate cause for his departure from Geneva appears to have been one of his outbreaks of cynicism and accurate scholarship, since in 1579 he was called before the Council for having caused to be printed a document enumerating twenty errors made by the Professor of Philosophy (de la Faye) in one of his lectures. The latter was incensed and outraged at this criticism and disparagement of his views and learning, and the quarrel assumed unexpected magnitude, since Bruno, on his second appearance before the Consistory or supreme tribunal of the Church, denied the charges and called the ministers "pedagogues."

These gentlemen decided to refuse him communion unless he should confess and repent of his faults and make due apology. His acceptance of these conditions not being hearty enough to suit his judges, he was admonished and excluded from the communion. These steps lead to greater contrition on his part, and the ban of excommunication was withdrawn. This sentence of exclusion was the only one within the power of the Consistory to pass, but does not prove that Bruno had accepted the protestant faith, nor partaken of its communion. In fact at his trial he steadfastly denied this. It seemed however, to disgust him with Calvinism, against which thereafter he never ceased to inveigh. Later he contrasted it with Lutheranism which was far more tolerant, and still later gave him a heartier welcome. Calvin, it must be remembered, had written a polemic against Servetus, "in which it is shown to be lawful to coerce heretics by the sword." As between the council of Trent and Calvin it certainly must have been hard, in those days, to select either a faith, or an abiding place where that faith might be peaceably practiced. Doubtless Bruno's views concerning the philosophy of Aristotle conflicted with those of the church authorities, for Beza (Calvin's follower), had stated that they did not propose to swerve one particle from the opinions of that Greek philosopher, to whom, though of pagan origin, the Church, both Roman and Protestant, was for centuries so firmly bound. And so shaking the dust of Geneva from his feet he journeyed to Lyons, where he failed utterly to find occupation, and then on to Toulouse, where he remained about two years. Here he took a Doctorate in Theology in order to compete for a vacant chair.

To this he was elected by the students, as the custom then was in most of the scholia or universities. For two sessions he lectured on Aristotle. Had this University required of him that he should attend mass, as did some others, he could not have done so, owing to his excommunication; though just why exclusion from a Calvinistic academy should debar him from Catholic mass does not appear. Toulouse was a warm place for heretics; the burning of 14,000 of them at its capture will prove this. A few years (35) after he left it Vanini was burned for heretic notions. It is hardly to be believed that Bruno could pass two years or more here without controversies arising from his teaching. But his nominal reason for leaving, in 1581, and going to Paris, was the war then raging in Southern France, under Henry of Navarre. Before leaving Toulouse he completed his "Clavis Magna" or "Great Key," the last word- as he seemed to think- on the art of memory. Only one volume of this great work, which, in his peculiarly egotistical way, he said is "superlatively pregnant," was ever published, and that in England, the "'Sigillus Sigillorum." It must not be forgotten that it was on both teaching and practicing this art of memory that Bruno, throughout his career, prided himself. He was even not averse, at least at certain periods of his career, to the belief that he had some secret system for this purpose, or even received occult aid. But when summoned before Henry III, to whose ears had come his fame, and asked whether the memory he had and the art he professed were natural or due to magic, he proved that a good memory was a cultivated natural product. He then dedicated to the King a book on "The Art of Memory."

But this was shortly after his arrival in Paris, in 1581, where he quickly became famous. A course of thirty lectures on "The Thirty Divine Attributes" of St. Thomas Aquinas would have given him a chair, could he have attended mass. His residence in Paris was marked by an extraordinary literary activity. He published in succession De Umbris Idearum (Shadow of Ideas), dedicated to Henry III, (this included the Art of Memory just mentioned) Cantus Circaeus (Incantation of Circe) dedicated to Prince Henry; De Compendiosa Architectura et Complemento Artis Lulli (Compendious Architecture);

Candelaio (The Torchbearer); these all appeared in 1582. These varied greatly in character. The first was devoted to the metaphysics of the art of remembering, with an analysis of that faculty, and these second was given up to the same general topic. It was all obscure, hence perhaps its popularity. Brunnhofer says that it was "a convenient means of introducing Bruno to strange universities, gaining him favor with the great, or helping him out of pressing need of money. It was his exoteric philosophy with which he could carefully drape the philosophy of a religion hostile to the Church, and ride as a hobby horse in his unfruitful humors."

Nevertheless we must believe in his sincerity. The "Compendious Architecture" is the first of his works in which Bruno deals with the views of Raymond Lully, a "logical calculus and mnemonic scheme in one" (McIntyre) that had many imitators. For Lully Bruno seems to have the greatest regard, this appearing in many ways. Lully, by the way, was a Spanish scholastic and alchemist, who was born on one of the Balearic Islands In 1235. He went as a missionary to the Mahommedans, and spent much time In Asia and Africa. He figures largely In the history of the alchemists and as a practitioner of the occult. The "Torchbearer" was a work of very different character. It was described as a "Comedy" by one who described himself as "Academico di nulla academia, ditto il fastidlto: In tristitia hilaris, hilaritate tristis." It is essentially a satire on the predominant vices of pedantry, superstition and selfishness or sordid love. Though lacking in dramatic power it is regarded as second to nothing of its kind and time.

Its *dramatis personae* are personified types, not individuals. It was realistic even in its vulgarity, for obscenity was prevalent in the literature of those days. But in it Bruno struck at what seemed to him his greatest enemy, i. e. pedantry. There were at this time in Paris two great Universities, one the College de France, with liberal tendencies, and opposed to the Jesuits and all pedantry; the other the Sorbonne, for centuries the guardian of the Catholic faith, endowed with the right of censorship, which must have been exercised over Bruno's works. In which of these, though surely in one of them, Bruno was made an extraordinary lecturer history has failed to record. He must have offended both, since he was anxious to be taken back into the Church, yet was revolutionary in his teaching. More than thirty years later Nostitz, one of his pupils, paid tribute to his versatility and skill, saying "he was able to discourse impromptu on any suggested subject, to speak extensively and elaborately without preparation, so that he attracted many pupils and admirers in Paris." (McIntyre). But Bruno belonged to the literally peripatetic school, and in 1583 he forsook Paris for London, because as he says of "tumults," leaving it to the imagination whether these were civil or scholastic.

Elizabeth reigned at this time; her influence made England a harbor of safety for religious and other mental suspects. She had a penchant for Italians and their language; two of her physicians were Italians, and Florio was ever welcome at her court. To this court Bruno also was welcomed, and, basking for sometime in the sunshine of her regard and patronage, passed there the happiest portion of his unhappy life. Oxford was at that time the stronghold of Aristotelelianism. One of its statutes ordained that "Bachelors and Masters who did not follow Aristotle faithfully were liable to a fine of five shillings for every point of divergence, and for every fault committed against the Logic of the Organon." (McIntyre). In Oxford at this time, unfortunately, theology was the only live issue; of science as of real scholarship there was little or none. (Its predominant trait of those days is still, perhaps, its dominant feature today). To this university Bruno addressed a letter, couched in vainglorious and egotistical terms, craving permission to lecture there. This was not received with favor, while his doctrines met with small encouragement at this ancient seat of learning, which Bruno later stigmatized as the "widow of true science."

But opportunity was afforded him to dispute publicly

before a noble visitor In June, 1583, a Polish prince; one Alasco, for whom great public entertainment had been provided. His opponent, defeated by fifteen unanswerable syllogisms, resorted to scurrility and abuse. This public exhibition put an end to the lectures on the immortality of the soul which Bruno had been allowed to give, and he returned to London. Shortly after this he published his Cena (Ash Wednesday Supper) in which he ridiculed the Oxford doctors, saying among other things that they were much better acquainted with beer than with Greek. But he criticized too cynically and lost thereby in popularity. This led to the appearance of the Causa, a dialogue, In which he was less vindictive. He admitted in this that there was much in the old institution which was admirable; that it was even the first in Europe, that speculative philosophy first flourished there, and that thence, "the splendor of one of the noblest and rarest spheres of philosophy, In our times almost extinct, was diffused to all other academies in civilized lands." What he most condemned was the too great attention given to language and words while the realistics for which words stand were neglected. Doctors were easily made and doctorates too cheaply bought. His charge in brief was that they mistook the shadow for the substance; a charge even yet too commonly justified among the strongholds of theology and other speculative dogmas.

Returning to London after this experience Bruno went to live with Mauvissiere, the French Ambassador. While the English records make no mention of his presence it is yet quite certain that he was frequently at Court, and that men like Sydney, Greville, Temple and others were his frequent associates. But as the Ambassador's influence was on the wane, he was not equal to his great trust. At this time our philosopher spoke of himself as one "whom the foolish hate, the ignoble despise, whom the wise love, the learned admire," etc. (McIntyre). Of Queen Elizabeth he wrote in most fulsome phrases, such as she too dearly loved. Before his judges, a few years later, Bruno apologized for his exaggerated expressions concerning a Protestant ruler, claiming that when he spoke of her as "divine" he meant it not as a term of worship, but as an epithet like those which the ancients bestowed upon their rulers; claiming further that he knew he erred in thus praising a heretic.

Bruno published seven works In England. The first was '"Explicatio triginta Sigillorum"- the Thirty Seals thus explained being hints for acquiring, arranging and remembering all arts and sciences. To it was added his Sigillus Sigillorum for comparing and explaining all mental operations. Then came an Italian dialogue "La Cena de le Ceneri" or Ash Wednesday Supper. This was written in praise and extension of the Copernican theory. Indeed quite exceeding it in teaching the identity of matter, the infinity of the universe, the possibility of life on other spheres, with a painstaking attempt to show that these notions do not conflict with those of Mother Church. Next came "De Causa, Principio et Uno" (Cause, Principle and Unity). This treated of the immanence of spirit, the eternity of matter, the potential divinity of life, the origin of sin and death, and many other similar abstruse topics. It was followed by De l' Infinito Universo ed Mondi, with numerous reasons for believing the universe to be Infinite and full of Innumerable worlds, with the divine essence everywhere pervading. All these works appeared In 1583. In 1584 appeared his "Spacio de la Bestia Triofante" or Expulsion of the Triumphant Beast. In this prose poem Jupiter, repenting his errors, resolves to expel the many beasts that occupy his heavenly sphere- the constellations- and to substitute for them the virtues.

In the council of the gods convened by him many subjects are discussed, among them the history of religions, the contrasts between natural and revealed religions and the fundamental forms of morality. In this allegory Jupiter represents of course the human spirit; the Bear, the Scorpion, etc., are the vices to be expelled. Unfortunately the book was quite generally regarded as attack upon the Church or the Pope, though what he really struck at was the credulity of mankind. It was dedicated to Sir Philip Sydney. Then came his "Cabala del Cavallo Pegasio" or Cabal, dedicated to a suppositious Bishop who was made to impersonate the spirit of Ignorance and sloth. It is a mordant satire on Asinity, Including credulity and unquestioning faith. After this he dedicated another work to Sidney. "Degl' Heroici Furori" (Enthusiasms of the Noble), a collection of sonnets with prose commentaries, like Dante's Fita Nuova, touching on the love for spiritual beauty arising from that for physical beauty attaining a climax in a sort of ecstasy by union with the divine. These sonnets possess a very high literary value aside from their other interest.

When his ambassadorial patron was recalled Bruno probably returned to Paris with him, during the latter part of 1585. Here he spent a year amid constant turmoil and excitement, and at his own expense. Though he attempted reconciliation with the Church he was regarded as an apostate. He held one more public disputation in which he advanced one hundred and twenty theses against the teaching of the Sorbonne, his side being taken by its rival, the College de France. The outcome cannot have been brilliantly favorable, since he soon after left Paris, in June, 1586. The collection of charges above alluded to was published in Paris after Bruno's departure, and again in Wittenberg, under the title *"Excubitor"* (The Ambassador.)

It was an arraignment of the Aristotelelians, based on the words of that great master himself. Bruno claimed the same right to criticism Aristotle that the latter claimed to criticism his predecessors. In it Bruno says, "It is a poor mind that will think with the multitude because it is a multitude; truth is not altered by the opinions of the vulgar or the confirmation of the many"- and again- "it is more blessed to be wise in truth in face of opinion than to be wise in opinion in face of truth." (McIntyre, p. 50). In addition to this Bruno had also published, before leaving Paris, a commentary on the Physics of Aristotle.

Tarrying somewhat by the wayside Bruno reached

Wittenberg, where, in 1586, he matriculated at its University, Marburg having curtly rejected him. Describing him here McIntyre styles him the "Knight Errant of Philosophy." Here Lutheranism dominated the theological faculty, while the philosophical faculty was dominated by Calvinism; views concerning the person of Christ, the "Real Presence," and the doctrine of Predestination keeping them apart in spite of Melancthon's attempt to reunite the two factions. From the Lutheran party Bruno obtained permission to lecture, and so for two years he taught from the Organon of Aristotle, as well as the writings of Raymond Lulli. To the University senate he dedicated a work on Lulli, "De Lampade Combinatoria Lulliana," whose chief purpose was to teach one how to find "an indefinite number of propositions and middle terms for speaking and arguing." He regarded it as the only key to the Lullian writings, as well as a clue to a great many of the mysteries of the Pythagoreans and Cabalists. It was soon followed by "De Progressu et Lampade Venatoria Logicorum" intended to enable one to "dispute promptly and copiously on any subject."

But again fate compelled a change of residence, for the Calvanistic and Ducal party gained in political ascendancy, to which party Bruno, as a Copernican, would have appeared as a heretic. After delivering an eloquent address of farewell he moved on, his next abiding place being Prague, where Rudolph II, of Bohemia, was posing as the friend of all learned men. Here he already had friends at court, and here he introduced himself with another Lullian work. To the Emperor he next dedicated a work of iconoclastic type, "One hundred and sixty articles against the mathematicians and philosophers of the day." For this the Emperor granted him the sum of three hundred dollars, and in January, 1589, he shifted again to Helmstadt, in Brunswick, where he matriculated again in the then youngest of the German Universities. This had been founded only twelve years before by Duke Julius, who was extremely liberal in his views, and intended to found a model institution, in which theology should not play too dominant a part. But while he received here a certain recognition fate again sported with him, for the Duke died four months after his arrival. Bruno obtained permission to pronounce a funeral oration, desiring to express his gratitude to the memory of one who had opened such an institution, so free to all lovers of the Muses and to exiles like himself, who were here protected from the greedy maw of the Roman wolf, whereas in Italy he had been chained to a superstitious cult. It was full of allusions to the papal tyranny which was infecting the world with the rankest poison of ignorance and vice.

The fatuous simplicity and the worldly blindness which Bruno displayed, in ever setting foot inside of Italian or papal territory after the delivery of this Oratio Consolatoria, may in one way be appreciated but never understood or explained. Moreover he had made himself persona non grata as well to the Protestants, who were scarcely more liberal than the Catholics. It appears that the great Boethius, superintendent of the Church at Helmstadt, had acted both as judge and executioner, and publicly excommunicated Bruno without a hearing, since there is extant a letter appealing from his arbitrary judgment and malice. The grounds for this judgment were never made clear, since no attention was ever paid to the appeal; but inasmuch as Bruno never really joined the Protestant profession it must have been meant to inflict some species of social ostracism. Boethius had himself to be suppressed later. But Bruno, finding too many enemies, left for Frankfort in 1590, "in order to get two books printed."

These were his two great Latin Works, "De Minimo" and "De Immenso," the introduction to the latter being the "De Monade." He worked at these with his own hands. In the introduction to the former his publisher stated that before its final revision Bruno had been hurriedly called away by an unforeseen chance. This sudden departure may have been due to a refusal of the town Council to permit his residence there, or it may have been a call to Zurich, where he spent a few months with one Hainzel, who had a leaning toward the Black Arts. Bruno wrote for him "De Imaginum Compositione," a manual of his Art of Memory. In this Swiss city he also dictated a work "Summa Terminorum Metaphysicorum" which was not published until 1609, and then in Marburg. But Bruno returned to Frankfort in 1591, where he obtained permission to publish his De Minimo, This work was on the "three fold minimum and measurement, being the elements of three speculative and several practical sciences." This like the two next mentioned was a Latin poem, after the fashion of Lucretius. The De Monade Numero et Figura dealt with the Monad, and with the elements of a more esoteric science, while in the De Immenso et Innumerabilibus, the Immeasurable and Innumerable, he dealt with the Universe and the worlds.

These three poems contain Bruno's complete philosophy of God and Nature. While thus staying in Frankfort for the second time Bruno was invited by a young Venetian patrician to pay him a visit, and become his tutor in those arts in which the philosopher excelled. It was the most unfortunate event in Bruno's unhappy life when he accepted this apparently tempting invitation. Mocenigo, his host, was of good family, but shallow, vain, weak minded and dishonest, with the fashionable taste of his day for the black arts. It is quite possible that he was moreover the tool of the Inquisition, which had long desired to entrap Bruno. It is probable moreover that the latter quite failed to appreciate how unenviable he was regarded by that Church to which he still felt that he belonged. Furthermore Venice was then a Republic and free, and he longed for his beloved Italy again. En route to Venice he spent three months In Padua, teaching there and gathering around himself pupils, even in that short time. He had barely left it when Galileo was invited there to teach; as Riehl has said, "the creator of modern science following in the steps of its prophet."

Early in 1592 Bruno went to live in Mocenigo's house. Trouble soon began. Entirely apart in temperament and characteristics, they soon disagreed. The pupil was deeply disappointed at not acquiring that mastery over the secrets of nature for which he had hoped, and found that there was no quick way to acquire a retentive and replete memory. And so Mocenigo announced to his friend Ciotto, the bookseller, his intent to gain from Bruno all he could and then denounce him to the Holy Office. While others were thus conspiring against him Bruno was writing a work on "The Seven Liberal Arts" and on "Seven Other Inventive Arts," intending to present it to the Pope, hoping thus to obtain absolution and be released from the ban of excommunication.

When Bruno at last appreciated the dangers by which he was surrounded he announced his intent to go again to Frankfort to have some of his books printed, and so took his leave of Mocenigo. On the following day, in May, 1592, Bruno was seized by six men, using force, who locked him in an upper story of Mocenigo's house. The next day he was transferred to an underground cellar, and the following night to the prison of the Inquisition. May 23rd his former host denounced him, with a cunning and lying statement concerning some of his views and teachings. Thus he was reported as stating that Christ's miracles were only apparent, that He and the apostles were magicians, that the Catholic faith was full of blasphemies against God, that the Friars befouled the world and should not be allowed to preach, that they were asses, and the doctrines of the Church were asses' beliefs, etc. (McIntyre). This was followed two days later by a second denunciation in which Mocenigo went to a diabolical extreme of deceit and hypocrisy; stating that all the time he was entertaining Bruno he was promising himself to bring him before the Holy Office. Within forty-eight hours the Holy Tribunal met to consider the matter; before them appeared the book-sellers who had known Bruno in Zurich and Frankfort, and before them came Bruno in his own behalf, professing his entire willingness to tell the whole truth. Within a few days Mocenigo made yet another deposition, denouncing Bruno's statements about the infallible Church. On the following day Bruno was again heard in his own defense, and appealed to the famous and fallacious doctrine of two-fold truth, acknowledging that he had taught too much as a philosopher rather than as an honest man and Christian, and that he had based his teachings too much on sense and reason and not enough on faith- so specious had become his argument with the terrors of the Inquisition before him. He further claimed that his intent had been not to impugn the faith but to exalt philosophy. He then beautifully epitomized his own views, claiming that he believed in an infinite universe, in an infinite divine potency, holding it unworthy of an infinite power to create a finite world, when he could produce so vast an infinity; with Pythagoras he regarded this world as one of many stars- innumerable worlds. This universe he held to be governed by a universal providence, existent in two forms- one nature, the shadow or footprint of deity, the other the ineffable essence of God, always inexplicable. Concerning the triune Godhead he confessed certain philosophic doubts as well as concerning the use of the term "persons" in these distinctions, while he quoted St. Augustine to the same effect.

The miracles he had always believed to be divine and genuine; concerning the Holy Mass and the Transubstantiation he agreed with the Church. As the days went by he became the more insistent upon his orthodoxy. He condemned the heretic writings of Melancthon, Luther and Calvin, expressed respect for the writings of Lulli because of their philosophical bearings, while for St. Thomas Aquinas he had the most profound regard. Other counts in the indictment which he had to face were his doubts concerning the miracles, the sacraments and the incarnation, his praise of heretics and heretic princes and his familiarity with the magic arts. He finally made a formal solemn abjuration of all the errors he had ever committed, and the heresies he had ever uttered, or doubts expressed or believed, praying only that the Holy Office would receive him back into the Church where he might rest in peace. Further examinations were held and the earlier processes against him in Naples and Rome recalled. After this there was a period of apparent quiet save that he remained in prison. It is not known to what tortures he may have been subjected, but it is recorded that he knelt before his judges asking their pardon, and God's, for all his faults, and professed himself ready for any penance, apparently not yet realizing the fate in store for him.

A little later it transpired that the Sacred Congregation of the Supreme Tribunal of the Holy Office, in Rome, desired to assume all further responsibility for the process against so distinguished a heretic. Accordingly the machinery of the Church was put in motion to this end. Negotiations with the Venetian Republic, somewhat tedious and complicated, which need not detain us now, were at last concluded. January 7, 1503, the Venetian procurator reported of Bruno that "his faults were exceedingly grave in respect of heresies, though in other respects he was one of the most excellent and rarest natures, and of exquisite learning and knowledge," (McIntyre) but that the case was of unusual gravity, Bruno not a Venetian subject, the Pope most anxious, etc. It was then decided to remit him to the Tribunal of the Inquisition at Rome; whereat it is duly reported, the Pope was deeply gratified.

To Rome then he went and here he was lost, so far as documentary records go, for a period of six years. How to explain this fact and this apparent clemency has bothered the biographers not a little. Whether this time was spent in an examination of his voluminous writings, which would seem incredible, or whether the Dominicans labored so long to procure his more absolute recantation in order to prevent scandal in and reflection on their order, or whether Pope Clement himself regarded kindly- in some degree- the great scholar who was so anxious to dedicate to him a magnum opus- to these queries history answereth not. The Dominicans pretended- years later- to doubt if he ever had been put to death, or whether he had ever really belonged to their order.

These statements are too characteristic to provoke more

than a sad smile. Finally matters were hastened to an end by the efforts of Fathers Commisario and Bellarmino; the latter being the zealous bigot who decided that Copernicanism was a heresy, who later laid the indictment against Galileo. Through their machinations Bruno was, in February, 1599, decreed on eight counts as a dangerous heretic, who might still admit his heresies, and he was to be granted forty days in which to recant and repent. But this period was stretched out some ten months, until December, when it was reported that Bruno refused to recant, having nothing to take back. Among the Tribunal at this time was San Severino, fanatical, bitter because of his failure to secure the papacy, who had declared that St. Bartholomew's was "a glorious day, a day of joy for Catholics."

It was decided that the high officers of the Dominicans should make one last effort to compel or coax Bruno to abjure. This he declined to do, whereupon, January 20th, 1600, it was decreed that "further measures be proceeded to, servatis servandis, that sentence be passed, and that the said Friar Giordano be handed over to the secular authority." A few days later Bruno was degraded, excommunicated and handed over to the Governor of Rome, with the usual hypocritical recommendation to "mercy," and that he be punished "without effusion of blood," which meant of course burning at the stake. Bruno's reply to his judges deserves to be printed in letters of gold whenever it can be recorded- "Greater perhaps is your fear in pronouncing my sentence than mine in hearing it."

Let us spare ourselves a too minute account of his execution. Some reports are to the effect that his tongue was tied, because he refused to listen to the exhortations of those members of the Company of St. John the Beheaded, better known as the Brothers of the Misericordia, who accompanied the condemned to the scaffold or the stake, resorting to the most cruel methods in order to provoke at least some appearance of recantation or repentance during the last moments of life. Right here let it be said of Bruno that whatever may have been his weaknesses before the Inquisition at Venice, he stood firmly by his creed when put to the final test, and died an ideal martyr's death because his creed did not agree with that of his persecutors. And so terminated the life of one of Italy's greatest ornaments and scholars. The occasion had not then the importance we assign it now. The burning of a heretic was a frequent spectacle, and the year 1600 was the year of Jubilee, in which the death of one unbeliever more was but the incident of a day. He had himself foreseen it, saying, "Torches, fifty or a hundred, will not fall me, even though the march past be at mid-day, should it be my fate to die in Roman Catholic Country."

There remains yet to comment on his character and to analyze his views. The greatest blot upon the former is his attitude before the Venetian Tribunal. Here he was at first defiant, even polemical, strong in his asserted right to use the natural light of sense and reason. Under greater stress he modified this to one of absolute and indignant denial, and finally became submissive to the last degree, cringing and finally begging for pardon on bent knees. That this attitude changed with his better realization of his predicament is undeniable. Moreover what keen and sensitive natures may do under the influence of torture is never to be predicated. How many of us could resist the persuasiveness of the rack when it came to modifying our beliefs? But whatever may have been his weakness at that time, he completely rehabilitated himself before his end, for were not his ashes scattered to the winds as a token that he completely failed to recant? Surely no martyr to science or dogma ever died a more dignified death, for the edification or example of others. What shall be said of his persecutors and prosecutors? Let us here be charitable; let us be just. Have we yet that absolute knowledge of right and wrong which can enable us to pass final judgment on men of the past, their motives and actions? Moral perceptions are the product of the race, the age and the environment; they vary greatly with the times. There is no crime in or out of the Decalogue which has at all times and by all peoples been regarded as such. The Church during several centuries enjoyed a monopoly of wisdom or learning as well as of opportunities for acquiring them. Zealotry, bigotry, intolerance, fanaticism, were the natural products of such conditions.

So were cruelty and disregard of human life. Join the mind of a bigot to the body of one who knows not fear, and the result will be a Loyola, or a St. Louis of France, who held that the only argument a layman should engage in with a heretic should be a sword thrust through the body. If then heresy was a crime, punishable by a cruel death in all the capitals of Europe, let us blame less the men who were trained and grew up with these notions, but rather more the Church which preached them, whether Catholic or Protestant. Only if one of these really were, as it still claims to be, infallible, then what has become of its infallibility? Or if heresy be held still a crime then what shall we say of the Church's ethics? If one were God-given the other Is un-Christ-like. But no free thinker can engage In theological polemics, or with Jesuitical sophistries, without letting his reason excite his emotions; and when the emotions enter the door logic flies out of the window. Let us say then that Bruno was in some respects so far ahead of his day and generation that they understood him not. And yet he was a torch bearer, save at his own last funeral pyre, shedding forth a light which illumed the centuries to come, and helping to make the period of the Italian Renaissance one of the most important and glorious in the world's history.

If better known and more widely studied, he would be by English and American students placed on that pinnacle which he deserves in the Hall of Fame. What shall be said of Bruno as a philosopher? He, first of all men in the middle ages, taught that Nature was lovable and worthy of study. Loving her, trusting, confiding in her, he found himself at outs with all the mental processes of his fellow scholars. In this way the natural method was brought into direct opposition with the ponderously artificial and strained methods of his day. He held that our eyes were given us that we might open and look upward. "Seeing, I do not pretend not to see, nor fear to profess it openly," he says. His philosophy was rather a product of intuition than of ratiocination, which became his real religion, for which Catholicism was a cloak, because in those days one was compelled to wear a cloak or live but a short life, and that within prison walls. What the medieval church. Catholic and even Protestant, has to answer for, as to the suppression of truth and provocation of hypocrisy, is beyond the mensuration of man. For the argument from authority he had the greatest contempt, and herein he set the world of thinkers a valuable lesson.

"To believe with the many because they were many, was the mark of a slave," (McIntyre). Before Bacon, before Descrates, he saw the necessity of "first clearing the mind of all prejudice, all traditional beliefs that rest on authority." He thus begins one of his sonnets: "Oh, holy asininity! Oh, holy ignorance, holy folly and pious devotion; which alone makest souls so good that human wit and zeal can go no further," etc. By the independence of his mental processes he was thrown quite upon his own resources, and his nature, already dignified and reserved, was made more introspective and self-conscious. In this way he developed strains of vanity and egotism which led him at times to the bombastic self-laudation of a Paracelsus. He had nothing but disgust for the common people and the sort of scholars (pedants) whom they admired. The vulgar mind was more Influenced by sophisms, by appearance, by failure to distinguish between the shadow and the substance. Take but two or three of Bruno's conceptions:

"He perhaps first during the middle ages taught the transformation of lower into higher organisms, following the Greeks who first enunciated the doctrine of evolution, which It remained for Darwin and Wallace to edit and illustrate as that law of the organic continuity of life, which we call evolution. He further wrote of the human hand as a factor In the evolution of the human race. In a way which should have commended him to the author of the Bridgewater treatise. He wrote of the changes on the earth's surface brought about by natural processes, which have changed not only the external configuration of the same but the fate and destiny of nations; of the identity of matter throughout the universe; of the universal movement of matter. Long before Lessing he showed how myths may contain the germs of great truths, and should be regarded as indications thereof. In this way, he told us, the Bible was to be regarded, holding its more or less historical statements to be quite subordinate to its moral teachings.

When we realize how to such highly developed reasoning powers as Bruno possessed, were added a phenomenal memory, a tremendous power of assimilation, a developed imagination, a poetic nature, the gift of easy and accurate speech and a temperament easily excited to fervor in attack or defense, we may the better appreciate his dominating greatness as well as his trifling weakness; the former being entirely to his own credit while the latter are ascribed largely to the faults of his time, and the fact that he was really living far ahead of his day and generation. He was not only the forerunner of modern science, he was the prototype of the modern biblical critic, foreshadowing the modern higher criticism, albeit in veiled terms, and as a matter of esoteric teaching; because the biblical critic of those days was burned at the stake, while today he is barely ostracized by the shallow and narrow minded, with whom he has at best nothing mentally in common. So much have four centuries of labor and vicarious suffering accomplished for the emancipation of the human mind.

Bruno had a creed, but it was too simple for his times. He rejected certain orthodox dogmas, (e. g. the Trinity, the Immaculate Conception) which commend themselves still less to the emancipated and cultivated minds of today. He absolutely rejected authority, which was a step toward reason comparable to the freeing of the slaves or serfs. He evolved a theory of evolution from *a priori* concepts, which it remained for Darwin to complete and demonstrate. He believed in the natural history of religions. His motives were of the loftiest, though his methods were not always those of today. He believed that the essence of truth inhered in those differences which kept men apart, and still sever them. He believed the law of love and that it sprang from God, which is the Father of All, that it was in harmony with nature, and that by love we may be transformed into something of His likeness. As Bruno himself says- "This is the religion, above controversy or dispute, which I observe from the belief of my own mind, and from the custom of my fatherland and my race." (McIntyre, p. no).

And yet this sublime man was burned as a heretic I let us stop when we hereafter pass through the Campo dei Fiori, as I have done many a time, and take off our hats to the memory of this great man, who, while small in some human traits, yet was the greatest thinker in Italy during the sixteenth century, whose memory may help us to forget some of the hypocrisies and cant so generally prevalent during the age which and among the men who condemned him. Let us also thank God that there is no Tribunal of the Inquisition today, to pass misguided judgment upon us for having gone further than Bruno ever dreamed, though along the same lines, and to condemn us therefore to the Flames.

This paper has already been prolonged, perhaps tiresomely, nevertheless I cannot refrain from quoting a few paragraphs from that most versatile student of this period, Symonds, whose estimate of Bruno is as follows: (Renaissance in Italy; Catholic Reaction, II Chap. ix).

"Bruno appears before us as the man who most vitally and comprehensively grasped the leading tendencies of his age in their intellectual essence. He left behind him the medieval conception of an extra-mundane God, creating a finite world, of which this globe is the center, and the principal episode in the history of which is the series of events from the Fall, through the incarnation and crucifixion, to the Last Judgment. He substituted the conception of an ever-living, ever-acting, ever-self-effectuating God, immanent in an infinite universe, to the contemplation of whose attributes the mind of man ascends by the study of Nature and interrogation of his conscience.

"Bolder even than Copernicus, and nearer in his intuition to the truth, he denied that the universe had "flaming walls" or any walls at all. That "immaginata circonferenza", "quella margine immaginata del cielo," on which antique science and Christian theology alike reposed, was the object of his ceaseless satire, his oft-repeated polemic. What, then, rendered Bruno the precursor of modern thought in its various manifestations, was that he grasped the fundamental truth upon which modern science rests, and foresaw the conclusions which must be drawn from it. He speculated boldly, incoherently, vehemently; but he speculated with a clear conception of the universe, as we still apprehend it.

Through the course of three centuries we have been engaged in verifying the guesses, deepening, broadening and solidifying the hypotheses, which Bruno's extension of the Copernican theory, and his application of it to pure thought suggested to his penetrating and audacious intellect."

Bruno was convinced that religion in its higher essence would not sufferer from the new philosophy. Larger horizons extended before the human intellect. The soul expanded in more exhilarating regions than the old theologies had offered.

"Lift up thy light on us and on thine own,
O soul whose spirit on earth was as a rod
To scourge off priests, a sword to pierce their God,
A staff for man's free thought to walk alone,
A lamp to lead him far from shrine and throne
On ways untrodden where his fathers trod
Ere earth's heart withered at a high priest's nod.

THE EVIL EYE

And all men's mouths that made not prayer made moan.
From bonds and torments, and the ravening flame,
Surely thy spirit of sense rose up to greet
Lucretius, where such only spirits meet,
And walk with him apart till Shelley came
To make the heaven of heavens more heavenly sweet,
And mix with yours a third incorporate name."

THE EVIL EYE

VIII: STUDENT LIFE IN THE MIDDLE AGES

An Address given before the Chas. K. Mills Society of Students of the University of Pennsylvania, February 19, 1902. (Reprinted from the Univ. of Penna. Medical Bulletin, March, 1902.)

I assume that every university student of today realizes that his possibilities and his opportunities are better in every way than were those enjoyed by students of bygone times. I take it, also, that you would not be averse to listening to an account of the habits, the surroundings, the privileges, and the disadvantages which surrounded students at a time when universities were young and when customs in general, as well as manners, were very different from those of today. With all this in view, I shall ask your attention to a brief account of Student Life in the Middle Ages, with especial reference to that of the medical student. Measured by its results, the most priceless legacy of medieval times to mankind was the university system, which began in crude form and with an almost mythical origin, but which gradually took form and shape in consequence of many external forces. It represented an effort to "realize in concrete form an ideal of life in one of its aspects." Such ideals "pass into great historic forces by embodying themselves in institutions," as witness, for instance, the case of the Church of Rome. The use of words in our language has undergone many curious perversions. Take our word "bombast," for instance. Originally it was a name applied to the cotton plant. Then it was applied to any padding for garments which was made of cotton.

Later it was used as describing literary padding, as it were, as when one filled out an empty speech with unnecessary and long words, and, at last, it came to have the meaning which we now give it. So with the word "university.", "Universitas" In the original Latin meant simply a collection, a plurality, or an aggregation. It was almost synonymous with "collegium." By the beginning of the thirteenth century it was applied to corporations of masters or students and to other associated bodies, and implied an association of Individuals, not a place of meeting, nor even a collection of schools. If we were to be literal and consistent In our use of terms, for the place where such collections of men exercise scholastic functions the term should be "studium generate," meaning thereby a place, not where all things are studied, but where students come together from all directions.

Very few of the medieval studia possessed all the faculties of a modern university. Even Paris, in Its palmiest days, had no faculty of law. The name universitas implies a general invitation to students from all over the world to seek there a place for higher education from numerous masters or teachers. The three great studia of the thirteenth century were Paris, transcendent in theology and the arts; Bologna, where legal lore prevailed; and Salernum, where existed the greatest medical school of the world's history. In spite of the fact that these, like all the other stadia of the Middle Ages, were under the influence of the Church, from them sprang most of the inspiration that constituted the mainspring of medieval intellectual activity, although how baneful such influence could be may be illustrated by the Spanish- that is, the ultra-Catholic University of Salamanca, where not until one hundred years ago were they allowed to teach the Copernican system of astronomy.

Under the conditions existing during the Middle Ages, with relatively few institutions of advanced learning, and in the presence of that spirit which led men to travel long distances, and very widely out of the provinces, to the cities of the great scholia, or, as we call them now, universities, the most imperative common want was that of a common language; and so it happened that not only were the lectures all given in Latin, but that it was very commonly used for conversational purposes, and appears to have been almost a necessity of university life. Early in the history of the University of Paris a statute made the ability of the petitioner to state his case before the rector in Latin a test of his bona-fide studentship. This may perhaps, in some measure account for the barbarity of medieval Latin. Still, as the listener said about Wagner's music, "it may not have been as bad as it sounded," since the period of greatest ignorance of construction and rhetoric had passed away before the university era began. John Stuart Mill even praised the schoolmen of the Middle Ages for their inventive capacity in the chatter of technical terms. The Latin language, which was originally stiff and poor in vocabulary, became, in its employment by these medieval thinkers, much more flexible and expressive. It was the Ciceronian pedantry of the sixteenth and seventeenth centuries which killed off Latin as a living language. Felicity in Latin counted, then as now, as a mark of scholarship, and six hundred years ago a schoolmaster could come up to the university and, after performing some exercises and passing such an examination as the doctors of music do today, could write one hundred verses in Latin in praise of the university, and take his degree.

The boys who went to the universities learned their Latin at inferior grammar schools, often in university towns. These schools were mainly connected with cathedrals or churches, although, in the later Middle Ages, even the smallest towns had schools where a boy might learn to read and write at least the rudiments of ecclesiastical Latin. In those days not only were the clergy Latin scholars, but the bailiff of every manor kept his accounts in Latin, and a tutor even formed part of the establishment of a great noble or prelate who had either a family or pages in his care. In those good old days boys were accustomed to seek the university at the ages of thirteen to fifteen. A Paris statute required them to be at least fourteen, and naturally many were older. Many of these students were beneficed, and boys were canons or even rectors of parish churches. In this capacity they obtained leave of absence to study in the universities, and so it was quite common at one time for rectors and ecclesiastics of all ages to appear in the role of university students. At the close of the fourteenth century, in the University of Prague, in the law school alone there appeared on the list of students one bishop, the abbot, nine archdeacons, 290 canons, 187 rectors, and still other minor ecclesiastics. At one time in the University of Bologna, in the registry of German corps, more than half the students were church dignitaries. Sad to relate, many of these clerical students were among the most disorderly and troublesome of the academic population, the statutes vainly prescribing that they should sit "as quiet as girls;" while, as Rashdall says, "even spiritual thunders had at times to be invoked to prevent them from shouting, playing, and interrupting."

Considering the youthfulness of what we may call the freshmen, as many of them went up to the universities at the early age already mentioned, it is not strange that we hear of "fetchers" or "carriers" or "bryngers," who were detailed to escort them home; but we must remember that the roads were dangerous in those days, and that protection of some kind was necessary even for men. Proclamations against bearing arms usually made exceptions in favor of students traveling to or from the university. Students, many of them, lived in halls, or, as we would say now, dormitories, and one of them assumed the role of principal, or was delegated to exercise certain authority. Quite often this was the man who made himself responsible for the rent, whose authority came only from the voluntary consent of his fellow-students, or who was elected by them.

When it came to the matter of discipline, the good old-fashioned birchen rod was not an unknown factor in university government. There seems to have been always a certain relationship between classic studies and corporal punishment. In medieval university records allusions to this relationship began about the fifteenth century. In Paris, about this time, when there were so many disgraceful factional fights, the rectors and proctors had occasionally to go to the colleges and halls and personally superintend the chastisement of the young rioters. We find also in the history of the University of Louvain that flogging was at one time ordered by the Faculty of Arts for homicide or other grave outrages. It is worth while to recall for a moment how grave offenses were dealt with in those days. At the University of Ingolstadt one student killed another in a drunken quarrel, and was punished by the university by the confiscation of his scholastic effects and garments, but he was not even expelled. At Prague a certain Master of Arts assisted in cutting the throat of a friar bishop, and was actually expelled for the deed. In those days drunkenness was rarely treated as a university offense.

The penalties which were inflicted for the gravest outrages and immoralities were for the greater part puerile in the extreme. In most serious cases excommunication or imprisonment were the penalties, while lesser offenses were punished by postponement of degree, expulsion from the college, temporary banishment from a university town, or by fines. In Leipzig, in 1439, the fine of ten new groschen was provided for the offense of lifting a stone or missile with a view of throwing it at a master, but not actually throwing it; whereas the act of throwing and missing increased the penalty to eight florins, while successful marksmanship was still more expensive. Later statutes made distinction between hitting without wounding and wounding without mutilation, expulsion being the penalty for actual mutilation. With the beginning of the sixteenth century the practice of flogging the very poorest students appears to have been introduced. During these Middle Ages they had a peculiar fashion of expiating even grave offenses. For example, at the Sorbonne, if a fellow should assault or cruelly beat a servant he was fined a measure of good wine- not for the benefit of the servant, but for all the culprit's fellow-students.

Those were the days, too, when trifling lapses incurred each its own penalty. A doctor of divinity was fined a quart of wine for picking a pear off a tree in the college garden or forgetting to shut the chapel door. Clerks were fined for being very drunk and committing insolences when in that condition. The head cook was fined for not putting salt in the soup. Most of these fines being in the shape of liquors or wines, I imagine that the practice was more general because the penalty was shared in by all who were near. With lapse of time the statutes of the German universities gradually grew stricter until they became very minute and restrictive in the matter of unacademic pleasures. A visit to the tavern, or even to the kitchen of the college or hall, became a university offense. There were statutes against swearing, against games of chance, walking abroad without a companion, being out after eight in the winter or nine in the summer, making odious comparisons of country to country, etc. This was particularly true of the English universities, where a definite penalty was imposed for every offense, ranging from a quarter of a penny for not speaking Latin to six shillings eight pence for assault with effusion of blood.

The matter of constantly speaking Latin led to a system of espionage, by which a secret system of spies, called "lupi" or wolves, was arranged; these were to inform against the "vulgarisantes" or those offenders who persisted in speaking in their mother tongue. It was the students of those days who set the example and the fashion of initiating, or, as we would say now, of hazing the newcomers. This custom of initiation, in one form or another, seems to have an almost hoary antiquity. As Rashdall puts it, three deeply rooted instincts of human nature combine to put the custom almost beyond suppression. It satisfies alike the bullying instinct, the social instinct, and the desire to find at once the excuse and the means for a carouse. In the days of which we are speaking the Bejaunus, which Is a corruption of the old French Bec-jaune (or yellow bill), as the academic fledgling was called, had to be bullied and coaxed and teased in order to be welcomed as a comrade, and finally his "jocund advent" had to be celebrated by a feast furnished at his own expense. A history of the process of initiating would furnish one of the most singular chapters in university records. At first there were several prohibitions against all hejaunia, for the unfortunate youth's limited purse ill afforded even the first year's expenses. As the years went by certain restrictions were imposed, and by the sixteenth century the *depositio cornuum* had become in the German universities a ceremony almost equal in importance to matriculation. The callow country youth was supposed to be a wild beast who must be deprived of his horns before he could be received into refined society in his new home. This constituted the depositio for which he was supposed to arrange with his new masters, at the same time begging them to keep expenses as low as possible. Soon after he matriculated he was visited in his room by two of the students, who would pretend to be investigating the source of an abominable odor.

This would be subsequently discovered to be due to the newcomer himself, whom they would take at first to be a wild boar, but later discovery to be that rare creature known as a bejaunus, a creature of whom they had heard, but which they had never seen. After chaffing comments about his general ferocious aspect it would be suggested, with marked sympathy, that his horns might be removed by operation, the so-called depositio. The victim's face would then be smeared with some preparation, and certain formalities would be gone through with- clipping his ears, removal of his tusks, etc. Finally, in fear lest the mock operation should be fatal, the patient would be shriven; one of the students, feigning himself a priest, would put his ear to the dying man's mouth and then repeat his confession. The boy was made to accuse himself of all sorts of enormities, and finally it was exacted as penance that he should provide a sumptuous banquet for his new masters and comrades. This latter ceremony consisted of a procession headed by a master in academic dress, followed by students in masquerading costume. Certain further operative procedures were then gone through with, the beast was finally dehorned and his nose held to the grindstone, while a little later his chin was adorned with a beard made of burnt cork, and his wounded sensibilities assuaged by a dose of salt and wine. All this constituted a peculiar German custom, although some means of extorting money or bothering those who were initiated was practically universal. In Germany this ceremony of depositio seems to have led later to the bullying and fagging of juniors by seniors, that gave rise to indignities while at the same time it more than exceeded in brutality anything of which we have read in the English grammar schools. These excesses reached their highest in the seventeenth century, and for a long time defied all efforts of both government and university authorities to suppress them.

In southern France this initiation assumed somewhat different form. Here the freshman was treated as a criminal, and had to be tried for and released by purgation from the consequences of his original sin. At Avignon this purgation of freshmen was made the primary purpose of a religious fraternity formed under ecclesiastical sanction, and with a chapel in the Dominican church. (Rashdall). The preamble of its constitution piously boasted that Its object was to put a stop to enormities, drunkenness and immorality, but its practices were at extreme variance with its avowed purposes. The matter of academical dress may interest for a moment. During the Middle Ages there was for the undergraduate nothing which could be properly called academic dress. In the Italian universities the students wore a long black garment known as a "cappa." In the Parisian universities every student was required by custom or statute to wear a tonsure and a clerical habit, such "indecent, dissolute, or secular" apparel as puffed sleeves, pointed shoes, colored boots, etc., being positively forbidden; and so the clothes of uniform color and material, like those worn in some of the English charitable schools, have been the result of the uniform dress of a particular color which medieval students were supposed to wear, and which indicated that at the time they were supposed to be clerks. At one time the so-called Queen's Men in Oxford University were required to wear bright red garments, and differences of color and ornament still survive in the undergraduate gowns of Cambridge.

While the students usually wore dark-hued material, the

higher officials of the universities wore more and more elaborate garments, until the rector appeared in violet or purple, perhaps with fur trimmings. The hoods, which are still worn today, were at one time made of lamb's wool or rabbit's fur, silk, such as those which we wear, coming in as a summer alternative at the end of the fourteenth century. The birretta, or square cap, with a tuft on the top, in lieu of the modern tassel on top of the square cap, was a distinctive badge of membership, while doctors and superior officers were distinguished by the red or violet color of their birrettas.

This so-called "philosophy of clothes" throws much light upon the relation of the Church to the universities, as well as on the use and misuse of the term "clericus." That a man was a clericus in the Middle Ages did not necessarily Imply that he had taken even the lowest grade of clerical orders. It simply implied that he was a clerk, I. e., a student. Even the wearing of a so-called clerical dress was rather in order that the wearer might enjoy exemption from secular courts and the privileges of the clerical order. The lowest of the people even took the clerical tonsure simply in order to get the benefit of clergy; and to become a clerk was at one time almost equivalent to taking out a license for the commission of murder or outrage with comparative immunity. Nevertheless, the relation between clerkship and minor orders is still quite obscure. It is quite evident that students of those days were not worked as hard as those of the present day.

Three lectures a day constituted a maximum of work of this kind, beside which there were disputations and "resumpciones," which seem to have corresponded very much to the quizzes of today, scholars being examined or catechized, sometimes even by the lecturer himself. Gradually supplementary lectures were introduced, but there was a period during which the university seemed to decline and decay rather than the reverse, when intellectual life was not nearly as active and studies not nearly as closely pursued. In the days of Thomas

THE EVIL EYE

Aquinas intellectual vigor was at its highest, but in the fifteenth century there was a distinct falling off. During these centuries, too, it was not unusual that students attended mass or religious services before going to lectures. This practice grew during the latter portion of the Middle Ages. Attendance was not, however, compulsory. Even at Oxford the statutes of the New College were the first which required daily attendance at mass. In those days lectures began at six in the morning in summer, and sometimes as late as seven in the winter mornings.

There is every reason to think that often lectures were given in the darkness preceding dawn, and even without artificial light. It should be said that these lectures were sometimes three hours in duration, and hence it might appear that three such lectures a day were about all that could be expected of a student. The standard of living for the medieval student was not always so bad as has been sometimes represented. University students then, as now, were recruited from the highest as well as the poorest social classes, and the young sons of princely families often had about them quite an establishment. At the lower end of the university social ladder was the poor scholar who was reduced to begging for his living or becoming a servant in one of the colleges. In Vienna and elsewhere there were halls whose inmates were regularly sent out to beg, the proceeds of their mendicancy being placed in a common chest. Very poor scholars were often granted licenses to beg by the chancellor. This was not regarded as a particular degradation, however, because the example of the friars had made begging comparatively respectable.

Those who would have been ashamed to work hard were not ashamed to beg. This custom, for that matter, is by no means yet abandoned. When I was first studying in Vienna, in 1882, I remember a young German nobleman who was reduced to such an extent that he lived absolutely on the charity of others. He kept a little book in which he had it set down that on such a day such a person had promised to give him so much toward his support, and he called regularly on his list of supporters, and almost daily, in order that the gulden which they had promised him might be forthcoming. There is the good old story you know, also, of the three students who were so poor that they had but one cappa or gown between them, in which they took turns to go to lectures. In the small university towns, where thousands of students gathered together during a part of the year- where means of carrying food were scanty, and food itself not abundant- it is not strange that student fare was often of the most meager sort.

The matter of food was not the only hardship of student life in those days about which we are talking. At that time such a thing as a fire in a lecture-room was unknown, there being no source of warmth or comfort, save, perhaps, straw or rushes upon the floor. The winter in the northern university towns must have been severe, but it is not likely that either in the lecture-room or in his own apartments did the student have any comfort from heat. This was true to such an extent that they often sought the kitchens for comfort. In Germany it was even one of the duties of the head of the college to inspect the college-rooms lest the occupants should have supplied themselves with some source of heat. In some places, however, there was a common hall or combination room in which a fire was built in cold weather. You must remember, also, that glass windows were an exceptional luxury until toward the close of the period under discussion. In Padua the windows of the schools were made of linen. In 1643 a glass window was for the first time introduced into the Theological School at Prague. In 1600 the rooms inhabited by some of the junior fellows at Cambridge were still unprovided with glass windows. Add to these hardships the relative expense of lights, when the average price of candles was nearly two pence per pound, and you will see that the poorest student could not afford to study by artificial light. Some of the senior students may have had bedsteads, but the younger students slept mostly upon the floor. In some places there were cisterns or troughs of lead, or occasionally pitchers and bowls were provided, but usually the student had to resort to the public lavatory in the hall.

Along with these hardships consider the amusements of this period, which were for the greater part conspicuous by their absence. Statutes concerning amusements were often more stringent than those concerning crime or vice. These were essentially military times, and tournaments, hunting, and hawking, which were enjoyed by the upper social classes, were considered too expensive and distracting for university students, and were consequently forbidden. "Mortification of the flesh" was the cry of those days, as even now among some religious fanatics. Even playing with a ball or bat was at times forbidden, along with other "insolent games." A statute of the sixteenth century speaks of tennis and fives as among "indecent games" whose introduction would create scandal in and against the college. Games of chance and playing for money were also forbidden; nevertheless, they were more or less practiced. Even chess enjoyed a bad reputation among the medieval moralists, and was characterized by a certain bishop of Winchester as a "noxious, inordinate, and unhonest game." Dancing was rather a favorite amusement, but was repressed as far as possible, since the celebrated William of Wykeham found it necessary to prohibit dancing and jumping in the chapel. Apparently, then, in those days a good student amused himself little, if at all, and had to find his relaxation in the frequent interruptions caused by church holidays. At St. Andrew's, in Scotland, however, two days' holiday was allowed at carnival time expressly for cock-fighting. On the evenings of festival days entertainments were occasionally provided by strolling players, jesters, or mountebanks, who were largely patronized by students.

Altogether, it is not strange that students in those days fell into dissolute habits, many having to be expelled or punished. We can even understand how some of them actually turned highwaymen and waylaid their more peaceful brothers as they approached the universities with money for the ensuing season. In the archives of the University of Leipzig there are standard forms of proclamation against even such boyish follies as pea-shooting, destruction of trees and crops, throwing water out of the window upon passers- by, shouting at night, wearing of disguises, interfering with a hangman in the execution of his duty, or attending exhibitions of wrestling, boxing, and the like.

Evidently, then, university life had its exceedingly wild side. One needs only to recall the history of the famous Latin Quarter in Paris to be convinced of this. This was the students' quarter in the old city of Paris as extended by Philip Augustus across the river. Paris then was surrounded by a cordon of monasteries, whose abbots exercised jurisdiction over their surrounding districts. Just to the west of the student quarter stood the great Abbey of St. Germain. Between the monks of this monastery and the students there were frequent conflicts, and it is recorded that in 1278, for instance, a pitched battle occurred between the monks, under their provost, on one side, and the unarmed and defenseless boys and masters, on the other, during which many were badly wounded, and some mortally. The matter was finally carried to court, and the monks were required to perform certain penances and to pay certain fines. Their brutality, however, was not effectually suppressed. In 1304 the Provost of Paris hanged and gibbeted a student, and was punished therefore by the king; while the subsequent history of Paris is one of constant conflict between students and the clerical orders. On the other hand, the clerical tonsure in which the Parisian scholar clothed himself enabled him to indulge in all kinds of crime, without fear of that summary execution which would have been his fate had he been merely an ordinary beggar.

Bibulousness was another striking characteristic of medieval university life. In those days they knew not tea nor coffee nor tobacco, but spirituous liquors in some form were far from unknown to them. No important event of life could be transacted without its drinking accompaniment. At all exercises, public or private, wine was freely provided, and many of the feasts and festivals which began with mass were concluded with a drunken orgy.

You have observed that so far I have made frequent mention of clerical matters. In truth, in northern Europe the Church included practically all the learned professions. Including the civil servants of the government, the physicians, architects, secular lawyers, diplomatists, and secretaries, who were all ecclesiastics. It is true that in order to be a "clerk" it was not really necessary to take even minor orders, but it was so easy for a king or bishop to reward his physician, his lawyer, or his secretary by a monastic office rather than by a large salary, that the average student, at least in the larger places, looked to holy orders as his eventual destination. How much of insincerity and hypocrisy there were among those reverend gentlemen thus constituted you may imagine better than I can picture. The Reformation, as well as the increasing corruption of the monastic orders, brought about changes which were not rapid, but which became almost complete, and led finally to the partial restoration of the ancient dignity of the early Church.

Without pursuing this part of the subject further, it may be imagined what a general alteration and reformation in all branches of study, as well as in the general intellectual life of the people, the founding of the universites accomplished. For the greater part designed for the confirmation of the faith, they often brought about a reaction against it. Like the other integral portions of the university, the medical departments of nearly all the medieval institutions came into existence through voluntary associations of physicians and would-be teachers. For a long time medicine was included under the general head of philosophy, whose standard-bearers were Aristotle and the Arabians. At Tubingen, in 1481, the medical student's days were divided about as follows: In the morning he studied Galen's Ars Medici, and in the afternoon Avicenna on Fever, During the second year, in the forenoon he studied Avicenna's Anatomy and Physiology, and in the afternoon the ninth book of Rhazes on Local Pathology. The forenoons of his third year were spent with the Aphorisms of Hippocrates, and in the afternoon he studied Galen.

If any text-book on surgery at all were used it was usually that of Avicenna. Some time was also given to the writings of some of the other Arabian physicians. At that time any man who had studied medicine for three years and attained the age of twenty one might assume the role of teacher if he saw fit, being compelled only, at first, to lecture upon the preparatory branches. He was at that time called a baccalaureus. After three years' further study he became a magister or doctor, although for the latter title a still further course of study was usually prescribed. The courses of medical instruction were quite stereotyped in form, and were carefully watched over by the Church. Nevertheless, it came about that the study of medicine once more was taken up by thinkers, although, unfortunately, not logical thinkers, whereas previously it had been almost entirely confined within the ranks of the clerics or clergy.

The most celebrated of all these medieval philosophers in science and medicine was Albert von Bollstaedt, usually known as Albertus Magnus, who died in 1280. His works which remain to us fill twenty one quarto volumes, in which he discussed both anatomical and physiological questions. It is exceedingly illustrative of the foolishly speculative vein in which many of these discussions were carried on, that they seriously discussed such questions as whether the removal of the rib from Adam's side, out of which Eve was formed, really caused Adam severe pain, and whether at the judgment day that loss of rib would be compensated by the insertion of another. Those were the days, also, when It was seriously discussed whether Adam or Eve ever had a navel. In spite of such follies, however, Albertus Magnus left an Impression upon scholarship In science. In a general way, which long outlasted him.

These were the days when the students organized themselves Into so-called "nations," whence arose that

155

conspicuous features of German university life of today of so-called students' Corps. These nations- each composed, for the main part, of men of one nationality- had their own meeting-places, their own property, etc. One of the principal means of instruction in those days was disputations, or, as we would say, debates, held between students, often of different nations, In which they were expected to prove their knowledge and mental alertness. When it is recalled that universities were larger- I. e., better attended- in those days than now. It will be seen to what an extent these nations were developed. Oxford, in 1340, is said to have had no less than 14,000 students; Paris about the same time had 12,000; and Bologna had some 10,000 students, the majority of whom were studying law.

The title of doctor came into vogue about the twelfth century. At first It was confined to teachers proper, and was bestowed upon the learned- i. e., those who had almost solely studied internal medicine, and who were required to take an oath to maintain the methods which had been taught them. For the title of doctor certain fees were paid, partly in money and partly in merchandise. The so-called presents consisted of gloves, clothes, hats, caps, etc. At Salernum it cost about $60 to graduate in this way, while at Paris the cost was sometimes as high as $1,000, and this at a time when money had much more purchasing value than It has today. It was then, as now, a peculiar feature of the English universities that but little systematic instruction in medical science was given. Just as the majority of English students at present study In London rather than at one of the great universities, so in those days did they go to Paris or Montpelier.

This win be perhaps as good a place as any to emphasize the fact that the clergy, having so long monopolized all learning and teaching, and having, at the same time, an abhorrence for the shedding of blood, which Indeed had been prohibited by many papal bulls and royal edicts, permitted the practice of the operative part of medicine- I. e., surgery- to fall into the hands of the most illiterate and incompetent men. Inasmuch as the Church prohibited the wearing of beards, and as many of the religious orders also shaved their heads, there were attached to every monastery and to every religious order a number of barbers, whose duty was to take care of the clergy in these respects. Thus into their hands was gradually committed the performance of any minor operation which involved the letting of blood, and from this, as a beginning. It came about that no really educated man concerned himself with the operations of surgery, but left them entirely to the illiterate servants of the Church. This is really the reason that the barbers for many centuries did nearly all the surgery, and why, at the same time, surgery fell into such general and wide-spread disrepute. From this it was only revived about one hundred years ago. Did time permit, this would be a most appropriate place to digress from the subject of this paper and rehearse to you the various stages in the evolution of the surgeon from the barber; but time does not permit it, and it constitutes a chapter in history by itself, which must be relegated to some other occasion.

It was about the beginning of the fifteenth century that the better class of physicians began to belong to the laity, and were called "physici" in contrast to the "clerici." Later they were known as "doctores." Until the fourteenth century most of them studied in Italian or French universities, the Germans even being compelled to go to these foreign institutions. In Paris they were required to take an oath that they would not join the surgeons. This regulation was founded as much upon spite and envy as upon any other motive. Many of the clerical physicians belonged to the lower class, and were so ignorant that even the Church itself was forced to declare many of their successes miracles. Although monks and the clergy in general had been frequently forbidden to practice medicine, the decrees to this effect were quite generally disregarded, except in the matter of surgical operations. In the ranks of the higher clergy, it must be said that well-educated physicians were occasionally found. There is, for instance, the record of a certain bishop of Basel, who was deputed to seek from Pope Clement V. an archbishopric for another person, but finding the Pope seriously ill, cured him, and received for himself in return the electorate of Mayence, which was perhaps one of the largest honorariums ever given to a physician. These were the days when magic, mingled with mystery, played no small role in the practice of medicine, and when disgusting and curious remedies were quite in vogue. Superstition and Ignorance everywhere played a most prominent part. For instance, it was, in those days, an excellent remedy to creep under the coffin of a saint. When a person was poisoned it was considered wise to hang him up by the feet and perhaps to gouge out one of his eyes, In order that the poison might run out. It should be noted that putting out the eyes was frightfully common in the Middle Ages, mainly as a matter of punishment.

It is said, for instance, that the Emperor Basil II. on one occasion put out the eyes of 15,000 Bulgarians, leaving one eye to one of every thousand, in order that he might lead his more unfortunate fellow-sufferers back to their ruler, who. It is said, at the sight of this outrage swooned and died in two days. It Is said, too, that this Is the reason why the Emperor Albrecht was one-eyed. What the revival of learning could thus and did accomplish under these conditions as above portrayed may be readily appreciated. The restoration of Greek literature, the revival of anatomy, the habit of independent observation- all told materially in this renaissance of medicine. The Italian universities became the objective point of all who desired a thorough medical education. The students chose the lecturers and officers of the university and had a large voice in the construction of the curriculum. The officers of their selection negotiated with those of the State, at least until the close of the sixteenth century. In spite of this general renaissance of medical learning and the impetus felt by the inspired few during the sixteenth century, it must be said that the general condition of medical science and of those who practiced it was not greatly improved. The superstition of the common people and the timidity and indolence of all concerned were about as marked as they have ever been in the history of human error, and the practice of medicine was at least a century behind the applied knowledge of the other arts and sciences. At that time the best physicians and doctors were to be found in the Italian universities, the French coming next, and, last of all, the German.

The Italian universities were the Mecca sought by those who desired the best education of the day, and of all the Italian medical faculties those of Bologna, Pisa, and Padua ranked highest. Those were the days, also, of the traveling scholars- a very marked feature of medieval life. They migrated from one of the Latin schools to another, and from one famous teacher to another, sometimes traveling alone, at other times In groups or bands, and practicing often the worst barbarities while en route, supporting themselves by begging and stealing. On their marches they stole almost everything which was not tightly fastened down, and prepared their food even in the open fields. The result was that most of them fell Into dissolute habits of life. A somewhat better class of vagrant students sang hymns before doors and received food as pay. Some earned money singing In the churches. They apparently both drank more beer and at less cost than at present. At that time the cost of beer was about one cent for a large glass. The younger students were called "schutzen," and, like apprentices In trades, were obliged to perform the most menial duties. The older students were known as the "bacchanten," and each bacchant was honored In proportion to the number of "schutzen" who waited upon him. When, however, this bacchant himself reached the university he was compelled to lay aside his rough clothing and rude manners and take an oath to behave himself.

Not only the students, however, wandered from place to place, but even the professors of the sixteenth century were nomadic, wandering from one university to another; for example, Vesalius, the great teacher of anatomy, taught in Padua, in Pisa, in Louvain, in Basel, in Augsburg, and in Spain. These habits may be partly accounted for by the fact that the students elected at least some of their teachers, and the professors who failed of re-election certainly may be considered to have had a motive for moving on. Salaries were certainly not large In those days. Melanchthon, the great theologian, received during his first eight years a salary of $43 per annum, and by strict economy was able during this period to buy his wife a new dress. During his later years his salary attained the sum of $170, which would be equivalent to $750 today. When Vesallus died his salary was $1,000 per annum, to which certain fees were added. It is not strange, therefore, that many of the professors pursued reputable occupations during their odd hours or that they took students to board. We hear today of frequent illustrations of the pursuit of knowledge under difficulty, but certainly during the ages to which I have referred the ardent student, were he undergraduate or professor, put up with an amount of hardship, meager fare, and trouble of all kinds which would stagger most of the young men of today.

Men were human then as now, and the universities were not above disputes and quarrels, which sometimes became very bitter and dishonorable, but were the indirect instrument of good, since they led in not a few instances to the founding of other universities. Thus, about the beginning of the sixteenth century, Pistorius and Pollich were both teachers In Leipzig, but holding antagonistic views regarding the nature of syphilis, became so embittered that they could not bear each other's presence, and each resolved to seek another home. The former influenced the elector to select Frankfort-on-the-Oder as the site of a new university, while the latter was the means of founding another at Wittenberg. It is pretty hard to keep away from the relation of the barber to the anatomist and surgeon when discussing this subject.

In another place I have dealt with the evolution of the surgeon from the barber, and have endeavored to show that the principal factor which operated to keep back the progress of surgery during the eighteen centuries previous to the last was the influence of the Church, which opposed the study of anatomy and degraded the practice of surgery. In the times to which I am referring now, an operation which caused the shedding of blood was considered beneath the dignity of an educated physician, and, in some circles, was regarded even as disreputable. It was, therefore, left to the only class of men who were supposed to know how to handle a knife or sharp instrument, i. e., the barbers. When operations were done in universities papal indulgences were often required, and these cost money, since in those days the Pope gave nothing for nothing. Public dissection required also papal indulgences, although in Strasburg, in 15 17, permission to dissect the body of an executed criminal was granted by the magistrates In spite of papal prohibition. The ceremonies attending demonstrations of this kind were both fantastic and amusing. A corpse was ordinarily regarded as disreputable, and had first to be made reputable by reading a decree to that effect from the chief magistrate or lord of the land, and then, by order of the University, stamping the body with the seal of the corporation. It was carried upon the cover of the box in which it had been transported into the anatomical hall, which cover, upon which it rested through the ceremonies, was taken back afterward to the executioner, who remained at some distance with his vehicle. If the corpse was that of one who had been beheaded, the head during the performance of these solemn ceremonies lay between its legs. After the completion of the ceremonies the occasion was graced with music by the city fifers, trumpeters, etc., or an entertainment was given by itinerant actors (Baas).

In time, however, this folly was given up, and by the latter half of the sixteenth century public anatomical theaters were established. The most celebrated was built by Fabricus ab Aquapendente, in Padua. It was so high, however, and so dark that dissections even in broad daylight could only be made visible by torchlight. The zeal with which gradually the better class of physicians pursued their scientific studies became more and more conspicuous, evidenced In many ways by the hardships with which some of them had to deal, as witness the struggles of many of the great anatomists of those days.

And so in time the clergy disappeared almost entirely from the ranks of public physicians, and after the Thirty Years' War completely lost their supremacy even in literary matters, this being gradually usurped by the nobility and the more educated laymen; but even then knowledge was pursued under difficulties, especially the study of anatomy. It was not until 1658 that a mounted skeleton could be found in Vienna. Strasburg obtained one in 1671. The handling of the dead body, which we regard as so necessary, was in those days avoided as much as possible. The professor of anatomy rarely, if ever, touched it himself, but he lectured or read a lecture while the actual dissection was done with a razor by a barber, under his supervision. Practical instruction in obstetrics, which would seem almost as important as that in anatomy, was not given in those days; male students only studied it theoretically. In the Hotel Dieu, in Paris, that part which was devoted to instruction in midwifery was closed against men. It was the midwives in those days who enjoyed the monopoly of this teaching, and upon whom the greatest dependence for obstetrical ability was placed. The physicians proper, or *medici puri* of the seventeenth century, were individuals of greatest dignity and profoundest gravity, who wore fur-trimmed robes, perukes, and carried swords, who considered it beneath them to do anything more than write prescriptions in the old Galenic fashion. Some continuation of this is seen in the distinction made even today in England between the physicians who enjoy the title of doctor and the surgeons who affect to disdain it. These old physicians knowing nothing of surgery, nevertheless demanded to be always consulted in surgical cases, claiming that only by this course could things go right. Still when elements of danger were introduced, as in treating the plague, they were glad enough to send the barber surgeons into the presence of the sick, whom they merely inspected through panes of glass. Very entertaining pictures could be furnished you illustrating the habits of the physicians of two or three hundred years ago in dealing with these contagious cases. The masks and armor which they wore and the precautions which they took would seem to indicate protection rather against the weapons of medieval warfare. At one time they were advised that if they must go into actual contact with these patients they should first repeat the Twenty-second Psalm. You may find in the old books, if you will hunt for them, curious pictures illustrating the precautions taken a few hundred years ago against the pestilence, of whose nature they knew nothing, and seeing them you may imagine the vague dread and even the abject fear which led the *physici puri* or physicians to send the barbers in to minister to plague-stricken patients, while they contented themselves with ministering at long range to their needs.

But gentlemen, I fear lest I weary you with a longer rehearsal of medieval customs and student follies. While they have all passed away some of them have survived either in tradition or in modified form, as will surely have occurred to you while they were rehearsed. You will not fail to note the steady progress of an ethical evolution which has toned down the barbarities and the asperities of the past, and which has substituted a far more ennobling life-purpose and method of its accomplishment than seemed to actuate your predecessors of long ago. It is small wonder that the students of those days bore an ill-repute with their surrounding neighbors. You may see better now, perhaps, why the medical student even of today has to contend with a prejudice against both his calling and himself, a prejudice begotten of the many debaucheries and misdeeds of his predecessors, and, I am sorry to say, even certain excesses of today. I do not know how I may more fittingly terminate these remarks than by reminding you that the profession which you students hope to enter has suffered most seriously In time past from the character of the men who have entered it, and that even today certain of Its members fail to have a proper regard for its dignity. It is axiomatic that those slights and indignities from which we often suffer, and the neglect and indifference of which we often complain, are in effect the result of our own shortcomings, and that we are ourselves largely to blame because of that which does not suit us. I beg you then to remember that even at the outset of student life there should be ever before you such an ideal of intellectual force and dignity, of power, of co-ordination of mind and body, as may keep you ever in the right way, so that when you at last attain your goal you may deserve that sort of benediction which I find in one of Beaumont and Fletcher's plays (Custom of the Country v. iv.):

> "So may you ever
> Be styled the 'Hands of Heaven,' Nature's restorers;
> Get wealth and honors, and, by your success
> In all your undertakings, propagate
> A great opinion in the world."

IX: A STUDY OF MEDICAL WORDS, DEEDS AND MEN

Study nature for facts; study lives of great men for inspiration how to use them.

Address in Medicine, delivered June 24, 1902, at Yale University Commencement. (Reprinted from the Yale Medical Journal, July, 1902.)

Never have I more earnestly craved the gift of eloquence than on occasions like this, when young men are about to leave the halls in which and the men with whom they have grown into man's estate, in order to assume the solemn and weighty responsibilities not only of their own lives but those as well of others. The day upon which you are thus released from duties of one kind to assume those of another, welcome and joyous though it may be, should nevertheless be interspersed with some serious and earnest thoughts and resolutions. Old Yale sets now her stamp upon you. It will prove a passport to many homes, but must never be abused. It will entitle you to the society of the cultivated and to the respect of scholars everywhere.

It will admit you to the ranks of the learned and cause you to be treated with respect and equality by some of the profoundest and most scholarly thinkers the world has even known. Yale has now furnished you with that which her ripe experience has shown to be requisite for young men commencing professional careers. As contrasted with the total of human knowledge its aggregate is not large, but it has not for centuries been the custom for men to grow gray in studies before undertaking to practice medicine, and when your own qualifications are compared with those which we of the passing generation possessed at the corresponding period of our lives, the comparison will furnish at the same time the most startling illustration of the rapid advance of medicine in the past twenty-five years.

THE EVIL EYE

Yale has always been eminent for the versatility and originality of her teachers. Her medical history has been so well told during the past year by one of her most honored sons. Dr. Welch, that it is not necessary nor wise to go now into such historical details. The trend of science today is along the lines of comparative investigation, and the Bible is by no means the only literary collection which today is being subjected to the "higher criticism." The inspiration claimed for the contributors to that great ancient Collection is denied to the writers of great modern works, where, nevertheless, fundamental truth is as requisite for the welfare of the body as in the other for that of the soul. Only by painstaking research, laboriously repeated, do we clear the old paths of the rubbish of centuries or discover totally new ones.

Pathfinders of this description have always abounded in this great Institution, drawn by common impulses or attracted by some centripetal force. And though it were perhaps invidious to mention names, I nevertheless must select two of Yale's great teachers whose names are still green in the memory of all men, and ask you to note how the examples they have set and the work they have done may furnish the line of thought in which I wish you to follow me for a little while. The science of comparative philology would seem to be far removed from that of medicine. Still, it is based upon an ultimate analysis of parts of speech, and men like Professor Whitney were, not only the comparative anatomists, but even the histologists- if I may use the phrase- of words. Comparative philology then is to medical terminology what embryology and comparative anatomy are to a study of the structure of the human body. The philologist loves to dissect words and trace them back through rudimentary stages and roots to their earliest forms. He loves also to study the evolution of an idea as conveyed by a word, and trace atavism or reversion in human speech.

Again you have here at Yale a wonderful collection of extinct animal remains restored with marvelous accuracy to semblance of their original form and appearance. The indefatigable industry and wonderful ability of Professor Marsh and his coworkers have enabled us to form ideographs of the living forms of earlier geologic ages upon this earth, which could not have been furnished had it not been for their remarkable knowledge of morphology and skill in synthesis. Indeed, where have powers of analysis and synthesis been more brilliantly displayed than by these men. It used to be said of Cuvier, the great French comparative anatomist, that if given a tooth from any beast, past or present, he could describe the animal and its habits as well as reconstruct his skeleton, so wonderfully are minute differences perpetuated, and so familiar was he with them.

Let us see, then, if it be possible to take some of our common medical words and by applying to them the methods of Whitney and of Marsh follow them back to their early forms and significances, and then construct from them ideographs of the customs, habits and superstitions of the men who used them. Such a plan systematically carried out might furnish both a fitting and a novel introduction to the history of medicine. Coleridge, you know, said we might often derive more useful knowledge from the history of a word than from the history of a campaign. Take, for instance, our word idiocy. The Greeks, especially the Athenians, were a race of politicians. Private citizens who cared little or naught for office were the *idiotai*, as distinguished from the public officials and office holders. It came about in time that men of such retiring habits and modest tastes were regarded as persons of degraded intellect and taste. And so the *idioti* were considered of inferior intellectual capacity. In other words, the idiot of those days was the man content with private life. How different from the present day when conditions seem so nearly reversed.

Our kindred word imbecile has also present reference to those of feeble, dwarfed or perverted intellect, and refers rather to mental than physical defects, though both must often be associated. But originally the lame and the deformed who were obliged to use artificial support, walked as it was said, in bacillum, upon a stick or crutch, and from this expression we derive our word imbecile. Let us trace, for instance, again, the etymology of our word palate. The Latin palatum is the same as balatum, that is, the bleating part. The ancient shepherds of the region of the Campagna watched the sheep as they went bleating (balatans) over those hills, one of which subsequently became the Palatine. Or take again our word mania. It is derived from unv- the moon, meaning the moon- sickness, and corresponds to lunacy from luna. You see the ancient superstition concerning the influence of the moon abides in the name. This brings up again the old ideas concerning the metal silver which was sacred alike to Diana and the moon, and consequently feminine in sex and attributes. Hence comes the medieval alchemistic term lunar caustic, and hence, too, comes its use in the treatment of epilepsy for which it was formerly much in use, since epilepsy was regarded as a form of mania caused by the evil influence of the moon.

By the way, this may also remind us of the peculiar views of the alchemists of the middle ages, who believed that the property of sex inhered in the metals. They believed, for example, that arsenic was masculine in sex, and so named it from arsen, male, and arsenikos, masculine. Medical, like comparative philology, is the more or less direct outcome of the earth's physical features as they have influenced the commingling of races and the conquest of nations. Medicine seems a science of Aryan parentage; in the Sanskrit the literature of medicine is rich; it was cultivated by the Greeks, but it lost much of its original significance by virtue of Roman supremacy, as the Latin races took it over. Under the Arabians it flourished after a fashion. With the revival of Greek learning there was a restoration of much that had been lost, but the supremacy of the Church kept it within extremely narrow limits, though the clericals could not eliminate all the Arabian words which had crept into Its terminology. Greek is today the language to which we turn for aid when it becomes necessary to invent new terms by which to indicate fresh discoveries or concepts.

The debt of medicine to our Aryan forefathers is great. Surgery was then a dignified branch of the science. Their autoplastic methods were conceived with great ingenuity and carried out with much, albeit with crude skill. The so-called Indian method of reconstructing a nose bears witness to their ability in plastic art. Their itinerant surgeons performed many capital operations; i. e., lithotomy and coellotomy. There is good reason to believe that Hippocrates knew nothing of practical anatomy, whereas, long before him Susruta urged that all physician priests should dissect the human body in order that they might know Its structure; and gave, moreover, directions for the selection of suitable subjects. The Sanskrit writers knew the properties of many plants and of at least five of the metals. Many Greek names of drugs are derived from the Sanskrit, or else they had a common Aryan origin. Thus the Greek equivalents for our words castor, musk, cardamon, chestnut, hemp, mace, pepper, sandal-wood, ginger, nerve, marrow, bone, heart, and head, are unmistakably of much older, I. e., Sanskrit or Aryan stock, several of them coming down In Romanized form, but almost unchanged- e.g., os, cor, moschus, cannabis, castorion. Although many of the ancient Greeks visited India, it appears that but relatively few words have come to us from this ancient source.

Our word sulfur, though, is of Sanskrit origin, the Greek work theion indicating its divine or god-given purifying power, with possible allusion to its utility in that lower world with which the theologians most often associate it. The Greek word appears in our chemical nomenclature as dithionic, trithlonic, etc. We note also an almost complete absence of Egyptian words, though many cultured Greeks visited Egypt. Nevertheless, the latter looked with small favor on barbarisms of speech, and our word pyramid is one of the very few which they thus adopted. The term surgery is of very distinct Greek origin, and meant handwork as distinguished from the action of internal remedies. Medicine seems to be derived from medeo to take care of, to provide, and physic and physician from *phusis,* i. e., nature. The physici were originally naturalists, or scientists, like Aristotle, medical science being but a part of their study. Campbell in his book ("The Language of Medicine") gives a list of at least two dozen common terms of today which were employed by Homer.

In addition to these, many other Homeric terms are still in use, but with more or less altered or perverted meanings; for example, aether, when used in the sense of its being a narcotic agency; astragalus, which originally meant a die, since the analogous bones of the sheep were used for dice; amoeba, from another, change or alteration, alluding to constant change of shape. Ammon originally meant a young lamb, iris a halo, meconium has reference to the juice of the poppy, from mekon, opium; molybdenum was so named from its resemblance to lead, narcosis originally meant numbness; the pleura was the side; the original phial was a saucer; the phalanges were so called because they were arranged side by side as it were in a phalanx; our troche was at first a wheel; and our tympanum was the original Greek drum, the word still persisting in musical terminology. The arteries were so named because they were supposed to contain air, while the veins were the gushers, from phleo, to gush or flow. The original confusion of nerves and tendons appears in the term aponeurosis.

Long ago there were two rival medical factions among the Greeks, the Empirics, from empeirikos, meaning experimental- who believed there were no philosophic underlying principles of medical science, and that experience alone was the safe guide- and the Methodists, from methodos, who believed it better to follow the hodos, or "middle of the road." The present use of the word empiric shows the contempt with which the former came to be regarded. As cure (euro) meant to care for, so did medicus have the same meaning, as already remarked, while the Greek slave, therapon, who waited on his master, became later the therapeutist who cared for his ailments. Our word to heal has also a somewhat similar dislocated meaning, since originally it meant protection, I. e., covering. The same root persists in hell, I. e., hades, referring to a certain supposititious locality so well covered that from it there is no escape. Note, too, the influence of ancient mythology in medical phraseology. Jupiter Ammon, the horned god, is recognized in hartshorn or ammonia. Mars, the god of war, whose symbol is iron, persists in the so-called martial preparations or ferruginous tonics.

Venus and Aphrodite naturally appear in venereal and aphrodisiac, while Vulcan's role is indicated in the heat to which caoutchouc is subjected in vulcanizing rubber. Mercury appears not only in Roman form as a metal, but in his Greek role as Hermes, not to be forgotten when receptacles are hermetically sealed. Let us cut short a longer list by simply noting in passing how the Greek Cupid Eros and his mate Psyche are perpetuated in our terms erotic and psychiatry, while Morpheus, the god of sleep, can never be forgotten so long as morphine is in use. That the wrath of the gods was to be dreaded is indicated in our word plague, from plege, meaning a blow from that source, that is their vengeance. You thus see the antiquity of the notion that epidemics were a divine visitation, and not due to bad sanitation. Melancholia, melas and chole, meant originally black bile. In ancient physiology the bile played a very important part, and the results of hepatic insufficiency were not only Indicated by this name, but the advantages of the use of calomel were amply emphasized by Its name, kalos and melas, for it was a beautiful remedy for this blackness. Another condition indicating trouble with the liver, which we call jaundice today (from the French jaunisse) was known as Icterus from ikteros, a yellow bird. The poultice which the average housewife of today Is so fond of using, was originally a pottos, or pudding, or perhaps a bean porridge.

In the days of ancient sacrifices one part of the animal was not placed upon the altar as an offering to delight the gods. It was that now known as the sacrum, which is usually defined to have been considered the sacred bone. The adjective sacer (sacrum), had not only the meaning generally ascribed to it, but meant also execrable, detestable, accursed. The sacrum meant then rather the part that was not acceptable to those to whom it was offered. The word calculus, like the term to calculate, must remind us of the presence of pebbles and their early use in facilitating reckoning, while our common terms testimony, testify, must necessarily recall the ancient sacred but phallic methods of oath-taking. Another superstition connected with deity is perpetuated in the term iliac passion, formerly applied to volvulus, or one form of acute bowel obstruction with its violent pain, which has been compared to that produced by the spear-point as part of the suffering upon the cross.

A keen analysis of the situation at the beginning of the Christian Era reveals the subtlety of the Greek character. The names of those organs which called for deep investigation or dissection are taken directly from the Greek, e. g., hepatic, sphenoid, ethmoid, the aorta, while many of the superficial parts have Latin names, c. g., temporal, frontal. It is to the Greek that all nations almost invariably turn when they seek to fashion new terms with which to characterize or name new discoveries. The Romans showed their appreciation of that which was good when they so readily adopted the science and learning of the Greeks, and were willing to take over even their gods. The Latin races have always been good imitators but poor originators, save perhaps in war and politics. Had they been willing to imitate the Greeks in these their history might have been very different. When the Latin translators of Greek medical literature lacked for a word they cheerfully took the original, sometimes giving it a Latin dress.

For instance, that which we now call the duodenum, meaning only twelve, was originally the dodekadaktulon, meaning that it was of a length equal to the width of twelve lingers, while they twisted the name eileon, the twisted intestine, into ileum. But the names of most diseases, like those of the more concealed parts, they copied almost exactly. While in later ages the Church completely dominated, then subordinated, and then finally almost terminated the study of the natural sciences, it is yet of no small interest to note the effect of the rise of Christianity upon the study of medicine. It has been well said that the same "cross which brought light to religion cast a gloom over philosophy" (Campbell).

Certain it is that the creed and the tenets which were for centuries the mainstay of Christianity, and which did so much for the uplifting of mankind, were made the excuse for the gradual suppression of all tendency toward investigation of natural phenomena, and the monasteries, where scholars congregated, became the graves of scientific thought and study. And so in time knowledge was exiled from Christian domiciles and transplanted to a Mohammedan environment. With Christian mythology and mysticism soon came also Christian demonology, and disease was generally regarded as an evidence of diabolical possession. This gave rise then, as even now, to the impostors who pretended to cure it by exorcism of evil spirits or invocation of divine or superhuman aid. It has always been a sorry time for rational medicine when superstition is rife. Even under the Arabians science flourished to but a limited extent. Their religion forbade the portrayal of any living object, animal or vegetable, consequently their works contained mere descriptions, never any illustration of any kind. This, by the way, is the explanation of their fondness for geometric tracery and of the richness of their ornamental designs. They professed the same horror of the dead body that was later inculcated by the Church and most of them scorned dissection. What wonder then that under Christianity and Islam alike our profession fared badly.

But very little now remains in our terminology to remind us of the period of Arabian supremacy. The Arabic words naphtha, sumach, alkali, alcohol, elixir and nucha (neck) are almost the only ones which have survived the renaissance. How different the monkish Latin sometimes is from the classic may appear In the use of the two words os and bucca for mouth, or os frontis and glabella for the frontal bone.

But this enumeration must not be prolonged unduly. Let us select three or four more examples almost at random and then pass on. But few will associate Christianity with cretinism. The early Christian inhabitants of the Pyrenees were known as Christaas, or in French, as today, as Chretiens. A mountainous region did for them what it has done in Switzerland for the races of today, and dwarfed the intellects of many while their thyroids underwent great enlargement. Such degenerates are known everywhere today as cretins, i. e.. Christians. Tarentum was the old Calabrian city later known as Tarento, where during the middle ages the dancing mania appeared in aggravated form. The frenzy was known in consequence as tarantism, while the spider whose bite was supposed to cause it was called tarantula, and a rapid dance music which alone would suit such rapid movements is still known as the tarantella.

Nightmare has reference to the old Norse deity or demigod Mara, who was supposed to strangle people during sleep. The Sardonic grin has reference to a tradition that in Sardinia was found a plant which when eaten caused people to laugh so violently that they died. But turn we now from words to those deeds which are reputed to proclaim yet more loudly the manner and the worth of their authors. Where may one look for a profession which shall afford greater opportunities? And where may he find one in which incentives are so small? The world's great rewards have been paid to the great destroyers of our race rather than to its saviors. Do you suppose that if Napoleon had saved as many lives as he lost he would have figured in history with his present luster? It is true that Lister's discovery has saved many more lives than Napoleon took. If so, the Hotel des Invalides should, when the time comes, contain Lister's monument and not that of a great murderer.

Personal courage is one of the noblest characteristics

which any man can display, particularly so when it combines the moral and the physical type. Public bravery brings nearly always its meed of public recognition. In fact, publicity is often the stimulus to a kind of bravery which without it would hardly respond to the tests. But your really courageous man is he who cares not for a search-light to reveal his deeds, one who dares and does within the quietude of his own environment that from which his weaker brothers would shrink. The soldier stirred to frenzy by the intensity of his passion will accomplish with but little dread that which might easily baffle the resolution of a reasoning man in a calm mood. The religious fanatic, be he Mussulman or Christian, may permit himself to be rent asunder rather than recant; but his motives are essentially selfish, since he looks forward to the Mohammedan's or the Christian's paradise, and so they are far from altruistic. But for that quiet heroism which shuns publicity, which calls for the highest quality of both mental and physical courage, which looks forward neither to the golden present nor the mystical yet sensuous future, commend me daily, yes hourly, to the sick rooms of patients suffering from diseases which menace the welfare of others, the infectious, the dangerous, the loathsome.

One may read of late many stories of army surgeons doing heroic deeds under lire, and one's heart naturally thrills with emotion as he imagines the scenes and wonders what manner of daring may lead a man to risk his life after this fashion. But I submit to you, that brave as is such a deed and worthy of all possible honor, it has been hundreds of times for one exceeded in the actual devotion to duty and the resolution required to brave the elements, or to face death elsewhere than on the battlefield, or to surrender strength or mayhaps life itself, or to invite disaster by infection, or to wear out and work out life in the constant grinding altruistic work of doing for others, who perhaps have violated every known sanitary law and forfeited their every right to live. Here is a theme that might well stir the most eloquent poet or orator that ever lived. How then shall I do it justice? Joanna Bailie has well put it: "The brave man is not he who feels no fear, For that were stupid and irrational; But he whose nobler soul its fear subdues, And bravely dares the danger Nature shrinks from."

This recognition of our profession was accorded much more unstintingly nearly two thousand years ago, at a time when it was much less deserved, when Cicero wrote (De Natura Deorum) "Homines ad inibus dando" (Men are never more godlike than when giving health to mankind).

But we can hardly delay longer here and at this time with the subject of heroism in medicine. I shall not have completed the matters which I wish to present to you today until I invite your attention to a short sketch of the careers of four or two of the men who, during the past two or three hundred years have set the example for men of all times and most climes, whose lives are so replete with that which is interesting, instructive or important that they may be well held up before a graduating class as illustrations of everything which may be advantageously imitated. They belong to that class of whom Longfellow wrote:

"Lives of great men all remind us
We can make our lives sublime."

One of those was Jean Fernel, who was born in France about 1497 and died in 1558. I do not know that his life history offers anything so very startling, although he came to be regarded as the most memorable physiologist of his generation, but he adopted a motto which I think we all might well select for our own, and it was because of this motto that I have mentioned his name at this point. It was this: "Destiny reserves for us repose enough." If each of you will take this Individually to himself he will find in it stimulus enough for all kinds of hard work. The first of the eminently great men now to be mentioned in this connection was Herman Boerhaave, born in 1668 and died in 1738. He enjoyed the reputation of being perhaps the most eminent physician who ever lived. The eldest son of a poor clergyman with a large family, he was originally intended for theology, and with this In view studied philosophy, history, logic, metaphysics, philology and mathematics, as well as theology. A mere accident, resulting from intense party spirit and doctrinal differences, prevented his devoting his life to theology, and he turned next to mathematics and then to chemistry and botany, subsequently studying anatomy and medicine.

He graduated in 1693 and began at once to practice in Leyden, with such success that he was early offered the position of ordinary surgeon to the king, which, however, he had the moral courage to decline. Subsequently he taught medicine and botany, to which chairs was also added later that of chemistry. This fact of itself will show to you something of the condition of medical science of that day, when one man could teach chemistry, botany and medicine. His rarest talents, however, were developed in the direction of clinical instruction, and in this particular field he won such repute that hearers were attracted to Leyden from all quarters of the world and in such numbers that no university lecture-room was large enough to contain them. His practice grew in extent and remunerativeness in pace with his reputation, and when he died he left an estate of two millions.

So famous was he that it is said of him that a Chinese official once sent to him a letter addressed simply "To the Most Famous Physician in Europe." That he had fixed convictions and practices may be better understood from the fact that so little difference did he make between his patients that he kept Peter the Great waiting over one night to see him, declining to regulate his visiting list by the means or position of his patients.

Boerhaave was universally regarded as a great student and a great physician, but it was probably his qualities as a man which led to the astonishing extent of his reputation. Essentially modest, not disputatious nor belligerent, he had a remarkable influence over the young men who came near him, while he had a habit of speaking oracularly or in aphorisms, which are not always so profound as they sound and yet often make a man's dicta celebrated. Save that he introduced the use of the thermometer and the ordinary lens in the examinations of his patients, his teachings do not form any really new system. In the classification of men he would be regarded as a great eclectic, in the purer sense of the term. Probably his greatest service to medicine was in the permanent establishment of the clinical method of Instruction, and perhaps his next greatest real claim to glory is the character of the instruction and the Inspiration which he gave to two of his greatest scholars, viz.:

Haller and Van Swieten. He was not the founder of a school. He left no great nor memorable doctrines for which others should contend, but he left a name for studiousness, honest and logical thinking, which was a priceless heritage for the university with which e was connected. The next great scholar to whose life and works I would invite your attention for a moment, is Morgagni, born in Italy in 1682, died in 1772. He was a pupil of Valsalva, whose assistant he became at the age of nineteen. Brought up in this way, as it were in the domain of anatomy, it is not strange that he devoted his attention throughout his life especially to the anatomical products of disease. It matters little to us now that he was wont to regard these products as the causes of disease and thus neglected their remote causes. He it was who taught us to apply to pathological anatomy the same scrupulous attention to tissue alterations and changes which the ordinary anatomist would note in dissecting a new animal form. He was scarcely the founder of the science of pathological anatomy, for this credit belongs to Benivleni, but he did very much to popularize the study and to show its importance. More than this, he wrote a work which for his day and generation was colossal. It bore the title "De Sedihus et Causis Morhorum per Anatomen Indagatis." It consisted of five books. The first appeared in Venice in 1761.

This proved a perfect mine of information to which one may often turn even today, and read with wonder the observations published one hundred and fifty years ago. They stamp Morgagni as a great scientist as well as anatomist. His industry will be indicated by the fact that even after he became blind he did not cease to work.

Perhaps the most wonderful figure in the whole history of modern medicine is that of Albrecht von Haller, of Berne, born 1708, died 1777, and often known as the Great. No more versatile genius than his has ever adorned our profession. A most precocious child, he developed remarkable abilities in the direction of poetry and music, as well as medicine, and the only wonder is that he lived to such a ripe old age, enjoying the fruits of his labors, having displayed throughout his entire life an industry and productiveness which were most remarkable. Before he reached the age of ten he had written a Chaldee grammar, a Greek and Hebrew vocabulary, and a large collection of Latin verses and biographies. During the next few years he translated many of the Latin authors, and wrote an original epic poem of some four thousand verses on the Swiss Confederacy.

All of this work he had completed by the age of twenty-one. It is not strange that among those who knew of his precocity he was generally known and regarded as a"Wonder child." It will thus be seen, too, that medicine was but one of the many subjects of his study. He studied a year in Tubingen, where the riotous living of his fellow students repelled him; then he went to Leyden, falling there under the influence of the illustrious Boerhaave. How much he drew from this source no man may accurately say at present, but a more brilliant example he certainly could not have had. He finished his studies In Leyden before he was twenty and then traveled through England and France, but was compelled to flee from Paris to escape arrest for hiding cadavers in his room for purposes of dissection. This will prove an evidence of taste for study if not of taste in other directions.

Suddenly developing a passion for mathematics, he went

to Basle and worked so hard as to almost ruin his health. This necessitated a trip to the mountains and here his interest in botany was aroused and indirectly that in medicine continued. Soon after he returned to Berne to take up the practice of medicine. Here he studied and worked so hard as to arouse a suspicion of his sanity, but he kept up his health by frequent trips to the Alps in search of flowers. His fondness for botany and his taste for poetry seemed to grow with equal pace and he seems to have been among the first of modern students to appreciate the beauty and grandeur of Swiss mountain scenery. When he was twenty-five years of age appeared the first edition of his poems, many editions appearing later. Here in Berne also he published so many essays on botany, anatomy and physiology that widespread attention was attracted to his eminent learning, and he was called to fill the chair of anatomy and botany in the new university of Gottingen, where he spent seventeen years of extraordinary mental activity, publishing countless papers and at the same time continuing his poetic and his nomadic habits. He established in Gottingen a great botanic garden, founded scientific societies, published five books on anatomy, all elaborately illustrated, printed a series of commentaries on Boerhaave's lectures, and is said to have contributed altogether thirteen thousand articles relating to almost every branch of human knowledge.

It is not strange that the fame of the University of Gottingen depended largely upon Haller's reputation. But Haller developed a clear case of nostalgia, and after being feted by the nobility, honored by almost every monarch in Europe, and receiving every honor that universities and philosophic societies confer, he resigned from his chair in Gottingen and returned to Berne, to his fatherland. Here, amid his old home surroundings, he worked for twenty years more at the same tremendous rate, discharging diverse duties of state and private citizenship, founding and promoting industries and asylums, and serving constantly upon commissions of all kinds. While thus engaged appeared that phenomenal work, his great Treatise on

THE EVIL EYE

Physiology, so full of original observations that it has been stated that should discoveries which have been re-discovered since Haller be collected they would fill several quarto volumes. The physiological institute of Berne is today known as the Hallerianum, as it should be, for it is distinctly the product of his genius. He died at a ripe age, after having performed an incredible amount of work, the greatest scholar of his own or perhaps of any century, revered and honored, faithful to the last and exhibiting in his last moments that "philosophic calmness of the cultivated intellect" of which Cicero loved to write. It is related of him that on his deathbed he kept his fingers on his own wrist, watching the ebbing away of his own existence and waiting for the last pulsation from his radial artery. Finally he exclaimed, "I no longer feel it," and then joined the great majority.

Perhaps Haller's greatest contribution to physiological lore was his doctrine of irritability of tissues. It took the place of much that had caused previous discussion and is accepted today as explaining, as nearly as we can explain, numerous phenomena. In this same great wonder-century lived also John Hunter, the greatest of England's medical students, the most famous surgeon of his day and the most indefatigable collector in natural history and natural science that ever lived. He was born In 1728 and died in 1783. He was led to study medicine by the fame of his illustrious brother William, and began his studies by acting as prosector for him. He soon became a pupil of Cheselden, perhaps the mast famous English surgeon of his generation. Hunter developed very early those extraordinary powers of observation and that originality in investigation which later made him so famous. Early in his medical career he came for a time under the influence of Percival Pott. This was at a time when surgery had emerged from barbarism and when the French Academy of Surgery had erected it Into the dignity of a science.

He entered St. George's Hospital in 1754 as a surgeon's pupil. Later he became a partner with his brother in the latter's private school of anatomy, but John, being a poor lecturer, was distinguished by his services in the dissecting-room rather than in the amphitheater. The customs of his time and the jealousies of the various medical factions then existing in London led to numerous acrimonious disputes, in the literary part of which William Hunter, who was much the more cultured student, took the lead, while John, who lacked in scholastic ability and had much less education, was relied on to supply the anatomical data. John was painfully aware of his deficiencies in literary culture and is said once to have replied to the disparaging remarks of an opponent: "He accuses me of not understanding the dead languages, but I could tell him that on the dead body which he never knew in any language living or dead."

It was in this way that he was led into unseemly encounters with the Munros, of Edinburgh, and with his late teacher, Pott. The same sort of dispute finally separated the two brothers, and they parted company after a very unseemly exhibition of jealousy and fraternal discord. After studying human anatomy for several years, John Hunter became profoundly impressed with the need for much larger knowledge of comparative anatomy, but about this time ill health compelled a temporary change and so he went into the army as a staff surgeon. This was at the time when Europe was engaged in the sanguinary Seven Years' War, and so it happened that Hunter had ample opportunity for studies and observations in military surgery- at the siege of Belleisle and later in the war in the Peninsula. Here he made many of those observations on gunshot wounds which he published at various periods later and which helped to make him famous. He resumed his work in London In 1763, and here again he had to undergo a long trial of those qualities of passive fortitude and active perseverance under difficulties which were his prominent characteristics. His personal needs were small but his scientific requirements were large, and to these latter he devoted every guinea which he could earn in his small but slowly growing practice. His own manners were so brusque, and he was so lacking in the refinement of many of his colleagues and competitors, that it took rare mental qualities to force him to the front, to which he nevertheless rapidly advanced. Bacon has said, "He that is only real had need of exceeding great parts of virtue, as the stone had need be rich that is set without foil," and this was never more true than in John Hunter's case. His leisure hours were never unemployed. He obtained the bodies of all animals dying in the public collections in London and so began to form that enormous collection which became known later as the Hunterian Museum. As his means afforded it he built and added to his accommodations and carried on those vast researches into animal anatomy and physiology to which the balance of his life was devoted. Although his practice gradually increased and he became in time the most famous surgeon and consultant in London, he used, nevertheless, to spend three or four hours every morning before breakfast in dissection of animals, and as much of the rest of the day as he could spare. Pupils and students who wished to consult him had to come early in the morning, often as early as four o'clock, in order to find him disengaged. He had that rare ability to do a maximum of work with a minimum of sleep which has been so conspicuous in the case of Virchow. Before he died. Hunter attained to a large competence, and his anatomical collection, consisting of some ten thousand preparations, made largely with his own hands, was purchased after his death by the Government, for seventy-five thousand dollars, and presented to the College of surgeons where it forms the chief part of the so-called Hunterian Museum.

Hunter's principal claims to greatness obtain in this, that he not only brought the light of physiology to bear upon the practice of our art, but by his writings and teachings and especially by his example led men to follow along the paths he cleared for them. It is no small claim to glory to be known by such pupils as Hunter had. By these, by his colossal industry in building up his museum, and by his writings, he will ever be known as the most prominent figure in the medical history of Great Britain. The fifth man in this quintet of geniuses which I am presenting to you today was Francis Xavier Bichat, who was born in France in 1771, and died in 1802. Although he was thirty-one years old at his death, his career was so phenomenal, almost meteoric, that it deserves to be held up as showing what one can do in the early period of his life, if he will but work. As one reads of his originality and talent one is led almost insensibly to compare them with those of some of the world's famous musicians who, also, have died in early manhood after giving to the world their immortal works, e. g., Schubert, Mozart and Mendelssohn. Bichat was the son of a physician and applied himself early to medical studies in Nantes, Lyons, Montpellier and finally in Paris, where he became the pupil and trusted friend of Desault, then the greatest Parisian surgeon. When Desault died, in 1795, this young man began lecturing for him, at the age of twenty-four. He displayed a wonderful, almost feverish scientific activity, more particularly in the direction of general and pathological anatomy. He was the originator of the phrase which he made famous: "Take away some fevers and nervous troubles, and all else belongs in the domain of pathological anatomy." Coming upon the stage shortly after Morgagni left it, he was able by his genius, his logical acumen and his graces of speech and manner, to give an attractiveness and importance to this subject which it had hitherto lacked.

It was his great service to more clearly differentiate closely related diseased conditions and to insist upon a study of post-mortem appearances in connection with previously observed clinical phenomena. He also established the tendency of similar tissues to similar anatomical lesions. In fact our view of what we call general tissue systems we in reality owe to him, since without use of the microscope he distinguished twenty-one kinds of tissue, which he studied under the head of general anatomy, while he held that descriptive anatomy had to do with their various combinations.

To Bischat was largely due the overthrow of purely speculative medicine because he placed facts far in advance of theories and ideas. Books he said are or should be merely "memoranda of facts." That he made many such memoranda will appear from the fact that before his untimely death he had published nine volumes of essays and treatises, nearly all bearing on the general subject of anatomy, normal and morbid. He also had not only his limitations but his faults. He strangely denied the applicability of so-called physical laws to body processes, he minimized the importance of therapeutics, and he sought to place the vitalistic system upon a realistic basis. Nevertheless he set an example not only for the young men of France, but of all times and climes, which should be often held up before them.

And so I have thus placed before you five bright and shining illustrations of what brains and application can accomplish, selected from different lands in order to show that medicine has no country, and from a previous century in order that you may the better realize how meager was their environment in those days as compared with that which you enjoy. Perhaps you will say, "there were giants in those days." True, but the race has not entirely died out. While Spencer and Virchow live one may not call the race extinct, nor can the times which have produced such men as Helmholtz, DuBois-Reymond, Darwin, Huxley, Leidy or Marsh, fail to still produce an occasional worthy successor. But it is time now to draw this rather rambling discourse to an end. The effort has been partly to attract your attention to some of the side lights by which the vista of your futures may be the more pleasantly illumined, and partly, by placing before you brief accounts of the careers of some of your illustrious predecessors, to show that eminence in medical science inheres in no particular nationality nor race, neither comes it of heredity nor by request. Like salvation it is available to all who fulfill the prerequisites. It is a composite product of application, direction, fervor in study, logical powers of mind, honesty of purpose, capability of observation, alertness to improve opportunities, all combined with that somewhat rare gift of tact, which last constitutes the so-called personal equation by which many humanitarian problems are solved. Study nature for facts; study lives of great men for inspiration how to use them,

> "Were a star quenched on high,
> For ages would its light,
> Still traveling downward from the sky,
> Shine on our mortal sight.
> So when a great man dies
> For years beyond our ken.
> The light he leaves behind him lies
> Upon the paths of men."

If then you regulate your mental habits by such a code other habits will of necessity fall into the proper line. The only other admonition I would give you in parting is summed up in these beautiful lines of our own Bryant:

> "So live that when thy summons comes to join
> The innumerable caravan which moves
> To that mysterious realm where each shall take
> His chamber in the silent halls of death,
> Thou go not like the quarry slave at night,
> Scourged to his dungeon, but sustained and soothed
> By an unfaltering trust, approach thy grave
> Like one who wraps the drapery of his couch
> About him and lies down to pleasant dreams."

That the sentiment is not new, however, will appear in this other and ancient version which Sir William Jones has thus rendered from the Persian:

> "On parent knees, a naked newborn child.
> Weeping thou satst while all around thee smiled.
> So live that, sinking to thy last long sleep,
> Calm mayst thou smile while all around thee weep."

IX: THE CAREER OF THE ARMY SURGEON

Commencement Address at the Army Medical School,
Washington, D. C, May 29, 1909- From "The Military Surgeon,"
July, 1909

The experience of listening to a so-called Commencement Address under these peculiar circumstances is doubtless as novel to you as is to me its preparation. So different is this occasion from that usually spoken of as Commencement Day, that it taxed my judgment as much as it did my ability to- as it were- "meet the indication," and to try to say the appropriate thing. It behooves me to remember that this is in effect not an address to a class of students just entering a learned profession, but an effort on the part of one on the borderland of experiences gathered from a civil surgeon's work, yet enjoying a quasi military title, with strong ties and leanings to some extent inherited- toward the course of the army surgeon and the fascinations of the soldier's life. Self-evident it is that you need no admonition which I could give, for the very fact of your presence here indicates that your selection by your superior officers stamps their approval of your ability as well as your character. Time has wrought vast changes in the personnel of the army medical corps, as in every other branch of the service. From the days of Xenophon, with his selection of the best material afforded, to the dark middle ages with practically no provision, then to the later centuries with their menial barbers and barber surgeons, and then the very gradually improved conditions which bettered the service, down to the present time, when the best is none too good, there has been that same evolution which has characterized all the rest of mankind's surroundings and man's realization of his public and private duties.

From the days when the first duty of the so-called army surgeon was to minister to his commanding general, and when the private soldier received but the scantiest if any attention, we have arrived at that time when the good health of the entire army is the aim and pride of the medical corps, and when public opinion demands for every enlisted man a degree of watchful care greater than many parents bestow upon their own families. The line officer of today can no longer afford to disregard the advice of his medical officers, and camp sanitation is now of even greater importance than operative technique, because preventable sickness and the incapacity caused by disease are recognized as far more to be dreaded than the bullets of the enemy. Public estimate of our duties to the sick and wounded has varied largely during different epochs. Thus Homer makes Nestor say:

> "A surgeon skilled our wounds to heal.
> Is more than armies to the public weal."

Homer also lauded the services of the two sons of Aesculapius, whom he deified as the grandest of heroes and the wisest of surgeons, and thus wrote of them at the siege of Troy, twelve hundred years before the birth of Christ:

> "Of two great surgeons, Podalirius stands
> This hour surrounded by the Trojan bands.
> And great Machaon, wounded, in his tent
> Now wants the succor which so oft he lent."

Again he thus describes an operation:

> "Patroclus cut the forky steel away;
> While in his hand a bitter root he pressed,
> The wound he washed and styptic juice infused;
> The closing flesh that instant ceased to glow,
> The wound to torture, and the blood to flow."

Contrast the tender mercies thus described with an incident occurring during one of the exciting experiences of

THE EVIL EYE

Ambroise Pare, who one day, during a battle, saw three desperately wounded soldiers placed with their backs against a wall. An old campaigner inquired, "Can those fellows get well", "No," answered Ambroise. Thereupon the old campaigner went up to them and cut all their throats, "sweetly and without wrath." Note, if you will, the expression, "sweetly and without wrath," since it implies a primitive form of humanity in providing euthanasia for the hopelessly wounded. While it has been from time immemorial the custom to attach surgeons to various armies, some idea of prevailing notions of antiquity may be gained from the statement that Xenophon had but eight field surgeons with his 10,000 troops. In his army the sick and wounded were cared for in adjoining villages, or, when on the march, were carried in the rear of the troops, being cared for by women from "the baggage." Whether these women were the "vivandieres" of those days I do not quite make out, nevertheless they must have been much the same thing.

In the days of Rome's greatest glory each cohort of 420 men had four surgeons, while each legion of ten cohorts had one legionary physician. In the navy there was also one physician to each trireme; nevertheless the wounded on land or sea received scant attention, although it is interesting to read that each soldier carried with him the most necessary bandages ready for use, an emergency packet supposed to be quite modern. A few hundred years later, in the Eastern Empire, the Emperor Maurice ordered that throughout every division of from two hundred to four hundred cavalry eight or ten of the strongest men be selected, in order to bring to the rear those who were severely wounded, to supply them with water, and to collect the weapons lying upon the field. These mounted cavalrymen received a small reward for each person rescued. Three hundred years later this arrangement was continued in operation by Leo VI. Wherever it was possible the sick and wounded soldiers were cared for by monks or by sisters, in the numerous hospices and institutions which abounded throughout the East, and although the care was often of the worst the efforts made were in the right direction. Holy oil, laying on of hands, supplication, and the use of holy relics constituted a large part of the treatment in vogue; nevertheless these remedies were not quite so injurious as some of the other and more disgusting ones whose use prevailed in those days.

Without doubt the two army surgeons who during the last 500 years achieved more fame than any of their colleagues were Ambroise Pare, and Baron Larrey. Such commanding figures were they, not only in their professional work, but in the general influence which they wielded alike upon sovereign and common soldier, that they will ever be regarded as among the most memorable characters of common history. Pare died in 1590, Larrey in 1842. Each was passed along from one ruler or commander to his successor, and each was regarded as about the most priceless legacy which could be thus transmitted. Parens name has always been most conspicuously mentioned in connection with the history of the introduction of the ligature as a substitute for the cautery iron or boiling oil, previously in use for the checking of hemorrhage, and for his teaching concerning the nature of gun-shot wounds, which had been previously and universally considered as necessarily poisoned wounds; but his new practice and his new views in these respects were but a small part of the general services which he rendered. It is not worth while to try to even epitomize here today the history of the ligature; though while its introduction has been widely credited to Pare, you must not forget that it was in use many centuries before his time, and was frequently mentioned by the early writers.

What Pare really did was, first, to abolish a barbarous and unscientific method of dealing with hemorrhage, and then to re-introduce or promote the employment of the ligature as a far preferable substitute, more humane, more clean, and more desirable. And so rather than do scant justice by incomplete reference to Pare's actual contributions to knowledge I prefer rather to speak of the other side of this great man's character, and to remind you of some of the many ways by which he secured such marvelous influence over those around him, and made his remarkable personality of the greatest use. As he passed through one campaign after another his reputation became more and more firmly established, and inspired surgeons the world over with the desire to visit him. In almost his every act his sagacity was conspicuously displayed, while, whenever they were called for, his personal courage and absolute lack of fear were equally apparent. Deprived of the benefits of early and liberal training he probably, on that very account, developed his power of thought, his memory and his analytical powers all the more keenly, inasmuch as these were made to take the place of what he might have learned from books.

The following anecdote will serve to illustrate, for instance, the general esteem in which he was held. In October, 1552, the army of Charles V. was besieging the city of Metz, and Charles himself came to take command. In the beleaguered city were gathered the nobility and the bluest blood of France, while at the head of the defending forces was the Duke of Guise. The imprisoned soldiers and civilians suffered alike from the onslaughts of the enemy, the rigors of a frightful winter, the lack of food, and the presence of disease. The Duke had established two hospitals for the soldiers, which he put in charge of the barber surgeons of the city, and furnished them with money with which to procure supplies, but owing to the wretched incompetence of these same barber surgeons nearly all the wounded perished, and the horrible suspicion arose that the soldiers were being poisoned. The Duke sent word to the King of France that the place could hold out for ten months, but that they needed more medicines. The King then sent for Pare, gave him money, ordered him to take all the medicines and other supplies he deemed necessary, and further aided him by bribing an Italian captain to permit the celebrated surgeon, in some way, to enter the besieged city. Braving all dangers, and being finally successful. Pare entered Metz two months later. He had at this time been with the armies for at least sixteen years, and was known by sight to officers and soldiers alike. On the day after his arrival the Duke of Guise dramatically presented him, on the ramparts, to all his officers, who embraced him, and hailed him with loud acclaim, while by the soldiers he was received with shouts of triumph. "We shall not die," they exclaimed, "even though wounded, for Pare is among us." The effect of this great surgeon's appearance was to give new vigor to the defenders, and to it was due the fact that the city was saved.

In his time Pare met with success such as today would be pronounced most extraordinary. He inspired the wounded with utmost confidence, and displayed, always and everywhere, remarkable firmness. Not the least notable feature in his personal history is it that he should have so long retained favor at court with such outspoken independence of character. Equally reputable among army surgeons of the past, and one of the most commanding figures in history, medical or other, was Baron Larrey. For more than fifty years he was an army surgeon, and for a great part of that period he stood really closer to Napoleon than almost any of the men whom the latter attached to his person by one or another of those traits that made him such a remarkable figure. That one of the greatest murderers and one of the greatest life-savers of all time should have been so closely drawn to each other, constitutes one of the most noteworthy incidents of history. Alike in many respects, so unlike in so many others. It is one of the most creditable features of Napoleon's career that he should have accorded to Larrey that recognition which he early gave and never withdrew. Never was such tribute more signally deserved nor worthily bestowed.

Though he passed through twenty-six campaigns, "from Syria to Portugal, and from Moscow to Madrid," and though his wonderful courage never failed him under the most trying surroundings of carnage and conflict, it may still be questioned whether it did not take a higher degree or order of courage to face Napoleon In his tent, or tell him plain truths in the Tullieries. The history of campaigning affords innumerable incidents illustrating heroism under fire, or equally trying circumstances, and it is difficult and perhaps unjust to single out a few for individual mention. Bravery is confined to no epoch and to no race; it is simply a God-given trait, not by any means possessed by all men. Take, for instance, one incident in the career of Larrey. During the landing of the English on the shores of Aboukir Bay, when General Silly had his knee crushed by a bullet, Larrey appreciated that immediate amputation was imperative, and gaining consent performed it, in three minutes, under the enemy's fire. Just as he was finished the English cavalry charged upon them; in his own words, "I had scarcely time," he said, "to take the wounded officer on my shoulders and carry him rapidly toward our army which was in full retreat. I spied a series of ditches across which I passed, while the enemy had to go around by a more circuitous route. Thus I had the happiness to reach the rear guard of our army before this corps of dragoons reached us. I arrived at Alexandria with this honorable, wounded officer, where I completed his cure."

Perhaps under no circumstance did Larrey's courage and zeal show to better advantage than in the awful retreat from Moscow. For example, after the terrible battle of Borodino, Larrey made two hundred amputations, practically with his own hands, where there were neither couches nor coverings of any kind, when the cold was so intense that the instruments often fell from the benumbed fingers of the surgeons, and when food consisted of horse flesh, cabbage stalks and a few potatoes. And all this while the savage Cossacks were hovering around equally ready to kill both surgeons and patients. Soon after came the passage of the Bereslna, with its attendant horrors. General Zayonchek, over sixty years of age, had his knee crushed, and was in need of immediate amputation, which Larrey performed under the enemy's fire, amid the falling snow, with no shelter except a cloak, held by two officers over the patient while the operation was being performed. The General recovered, and died fourteen years later as Viceroy of Poland.

It was after this passage of the Beresina by the Imperial

THE EVIL EYE

Guard that it was discovered that all the requisites for the sick and wounded had been left behind and on the other side. Larrey at once recrossed the river, and found himself amidst a furious, struggling crowd, in danger of being crushed to death, when suddenly the soldiers recognized him. Immediately they took him up in their arms, crossed the river with him, crying, "let us save him who saved us," and forgot their own safety in their regard for him whose merciful kindness they had so often experienced. Another incident in Larrey's career: Ever faithful to Napoleon, his adored master, through victory or reverse, Larrey stood one night with a small group of medical men gazing over the field of Waterloo, and upon the wounded and dying who lay groaning around him. Suddenly they were charged by a squadron of Prussian Lancers, at whom Larrey fired his pistols and galloped away, but was overtaken by the Prussians, who shot his horse, sabred him, and left him for dead. After a while he recovered his senses, and tried to make his way across lots to France, but was again captured by another detachment of cavalry, who robbed him of everything, and then took him to headquarters, where it was ordered that he be shot. Think of such a fate for one who had saved so many lives! But the order would have been carried out promptly had not one of the Prussian surgeons recognized Larrey, having attended his lectures several years previously. Accordingly he was brought before Billow, and finally before Marshall Blucher, whose son had been wounded and captured by the French in the Austrian Campaign, and whose life had been saved by Larrey's exertions.

You may imagine that it did not take long to reverse that order for execution. Praise from Napoleon was most rare, but of Larrey he made this remark in his will, along with a bequest of 100,000 francs, "He is the most virtuous man I have ever known."

Let us mention a few other instances. For example. Surgeon Thomson, who during the Crimean war, after the battle of the Alma, volunteered, with his servant, John McGrath, to remain behind on the open, unsheltered field, with five hundred Russians so wounded as to be disabled or even at at the point of death. For three days and nights these two Englishmen remained practically alone upon that field, covered only with dead and dying, among foreign foes, none of them able to help themselves, or even to speak in a language that could be understood. At the battle of Inkerman Assistant Surgeon Wolesley had established his field hospital in that awful place of slaughter, the Sandbag Battery. When its defenders were reduced to 150 men, and were forced to leave it, most of them retreated in one direction to find, only thirty paces away, a Russian battalion blocking their path. There was not one competent officer left, so this surgeon took command. Seizing a bayonet because he had no sword, he spoke hurriedly to the men, and explained that their next fight was not merely for victory, but for their own lives; then he led them in a charge that tore so fiercely through the Russian detachment that but half of them reached the other side alive. During the South African campaign the papers recorded (but how few read of it?) the fate of Surgeon Landon, who was shot through the spine while ministering to the wounded on Majuba Hill. Paralyzed below the waist, he had himself propped up, and continued his work as best he could until his strength failed, when he said, "I am dying; do what you can for the wounded."

It may be of interest to devote here a few minutes to the consideration of conditions obtaining at the time of our Revolutionary War. In 1776 the barber surgeon still had a place in the armies of the world and was even then regarded as scarcely more than a menial. Never was he accorded the respect or the honors of a gentleman, nor was he allowed to carry a sword. On the other hand, he was subjected to corporal punishment, and could be caned by his colonel, or almost anyone else, whenever such an act was provoked. It may be said that the English troops were somewhat better equipped than were the hired Hessians, while the French, who came to our aid, brought with them some far better men, who were in many respects a revelation during our revolution and an inspiration to our own so-called surgeons. But our colonial and general governments dealt very stingily with our army medical department, and their professional equipments were of the most meager; in fact, the history of surgery of those days, either in the army or in civil life, is practically the history of a few prominent individuals, most of whom had spent the time and money required for study abroad, and who had come home bringing back with them the best of their day, such as it was. For instance, there were the Warren brothers, in Boston, of whom the elder, Joseph, started Paul Revere on his famous ride. He was elected President of the Provincial Congress, and just before the battle of Bunker Hill was made Major General of the Continental forces, a position which he preferred to that of Physician General, which he had been offered. During the battle he fought with a musket, as though a private, and was shot down just as the conflict ended. The younger brother, John, lived to achieve fame and reputation, and transmitted them to his posterity.

During the war some colonial regiments even came into camp without any surgeon, or the slightest provision for disease or injury. In 1776 Congress ordered that there should be one surgeon and five assistants to each 5,000 enlisted men, the former being paid $1.66 per day, the latter $1 a day. Imagine the attention that could be bestowed upon 5,000 soldiers by six men whose services were thus compensated. Camp hygiene, hospital corps, and ambulance service were undreamed of; nevertheless John Warren, then only twenty-three years of age, accomplished a great deal in building up a medical corps, while as much more was done by Benjamin Church, of Boston, who was styled Director General and Chief Physician, and who was paid $4 a day.

Unfortunately Church was detected in traitorous correspondence with the enemy, was court-martialed, imprisoned for a year, then allowed to leave the country, and was probably lost at sea. He was succeeded by John Morgan, of Philadelphia, who had to fight the politicians as well as the foreign enemy and, failing to satisfy them, was dismissed from the service, though acquitted from all blame. Thus you see that even in those days the politicians made it hard to secure adequate and proper care for our sick and wounded soldiers. Everywhere at that time were unrest, excitement, and suspicion, and their demoralizing effects showed in every department of military as of civil government. After Morgan came Shippen, who held office from 1777 to 1781, under whose guidance affairs in the medical department improved very much. Smallpox had been perhaps the greatest scourge of the soldiers, as well as of the people in general, but this was kept in subjection by the practice of inoculation, which had been generally accepted in this country by nearly all men from Washington down.

A word or two must also be said about that remarkable man, Benjamin Rush, with his many-sided, versatile, erratic, obstinate and querulous character, who nevertheless constituted in his day the most prominent figure in the profession; who served two years in Congress; who signed the Declaration of independence; and who, in the same year, got his first army medical experience. It was perhaps not strange that, with his peculiar temperament, he failed to come under the influence of Washington's peculiar personal magnetism, and that their personal relations were not at all to Rush's credit, since he endeavored in many ways to belittle his Commander-in-Chief, and suffered therefor a rather ignominious exposure. The temptation is always to place most stress upon accounts of heroism which happens to be most publicly performed. While this is not unnatural it is often an injustice, since an act of courage may be performed in the lime-light of publicity, with a regard for notoriety, that would be lost were it done in private. It perhaps is not kind to think that anyone would ever be more courageous in public than in private, and yet it is to be feared that human nature is not always free from temptation of this kind. But the real silent heroes of military or civil medical life are those who engage in duties which nevertheless have even more of danger about them than spectacular performances upon the battle field. Take for instance, the work done by Major Reed and Dr. Carroll, who devoted themselves for months to the study of yellow fever. Many a man will stand upon the field of battle permitting himself to be fired upon, but how many will deliberately submit to being bitten by insects believed to be carriers of the germs of yellow fever. Dr. Carroll had this quiet kind of bravery, and allowed himself to be bitten by a mosquito that twelve days previously had filled himself with the blood of a yellow fever patient, and in consequence suffered from a severe attack, barely escaping with his life. Dr. Lazear permitted the same experiment upon himself, but was not at that time infected; but some days later while in the yellow fever ward he was bitten by a mosquito, made careful note of the fact, acquired the disease in its most hideous form, and died a martyr to science, as true a hero as ever died upon fortress or man-of-war. Others, too, willingly exposed themselves, but there was at that time no other fatality to record. But realizing the value of the service rendered, the indisputable proof of the nature of the disease, and the method by which it is carried, the value of the demonstration becomes inestimable, since a true prophylaxis was demonstrated, and a means furnished of ridding the community of this fearful pestilence. Moreover, it was shown how unnecessary it is to destroy valuable property, it being only necessary to kill the mosquitoes, and do away with their breeding places. Major Reed died a few years after he had led in this fight against the dread disease, but no monument, or other testimonial which can be erected to the memory of Reed, Carroll and Lazear can adequately express the value of the service which they have rendered to the world.

"Peace hath her victories no less than war." This epigram is as true of the conflicts in which the medical profession engage as of any other. This same sentiment has been put in other words. It is said, "That peace hath higher tests of manhood than battle ever knew." For instance, in New York there is a simple tablet commemorating, in loving remembrance, the death of eighteen young physicians who, one after another, attended a ship load of emigrants sick of typhus fever on Quarantine Island. They fought their good fight and were buried without martial music, adding eighteen names to the innumerable list of victims who have fought the silent battle of dealing with disease, public gainers only in this, that someone has been thoughtful enough to record their names in this semi-public fashion.

Taken again the case of Dr. Franz Muller, of Vienna, who contracted the bubonic plague while working in the laboratory with its germs. Just so soon as he realized that he himself was infected he locked himself in an isolated room, and pasted upon the window pane a sheet of paper containing this message, "I am suffering from plague. Do not send a doctor to me, as in any event my end will come in four or five days." He refused to admit those who were anxious to do for him, wrote a letter to his parents which he placed against the window, so that it could be copied from the outside, then burned the original, fearing that if sent through the mail it might carry the elusive germ. Was not this equal to any instance of valor under the excitement or the stress of battle and cannonade? Could anyone more worthily win a Victorian Cross, or any other emblem of courage and heroism?

Many of you have been in, or will go to Havana. It will be worth your while to make a pilgrimage to the cemetery there, where were buried sixteen young medical students who lost their lives under peculiar circumstances, which afford as well an illustration of Spanish tyranny and injustice. In 1871 one of the professors in the medical school died, and was followed to his grave by the students whom he had taught, and who loved him. Unfortunately they committed an indiscretion by scribbling with a pencil in a public place some criticism on the government; in consequence they were reported, arrested and court-martialed. The written paragraphs were evidence sufficient, and the Governor General ordered the ranks of students to be decimated. There were 160 students all told, and in accordance with this sentence sixteen of them were next day shot without any further ceremony. Of these the youngest was not quite sixteen years old, and his father offered his entire fortune for his life, but without avail. Later the citizens of Havana erected a monument of white marble, at no small cost, to commemorate this sacrifice.

here comes over me, as I prepare these words to read to you, a feeling of their inadequacy, and of lack of personal justice to many of my auditors. Brought up in civil life, with but a smattering of military training, I am rehearsing incidents of which you may read as easily as I, while at the same time I do not forget that from the lives of many of my auditors there might be drawn just as many illustrations of courage, fortitude, endurance and personal valor as any that the Surgeon General's library records. Unfortunately I am not familiar with them. They are, happily in one respect, too numerous to mention, and again are not yet public property, because modesty is ever the accompaniment of these other traits which we all admire so much. Hence, gentlemen, if I seem to you to disregard or forget many an incident in your lives or the careers of your friends, ascribe it to my ignorance rather than to my intent, and to the fact that I have never seen a battle, and that my fights with disease have not been fought in camps, but within the walls of the quiet sick room or hospital ward. Nevertheless I am never happier than when I can try to compel a wider public recognition of what you are constantly doing and of your valorous deeds.

Next to those general improvements In the service which have come about through natural causes, and as results of a better appreciation of its needs, and of a generally improved state of the profession, nothing has come from outside during the past fifty years which has been so helpful and advantageous as the support afforded by the Red Cross, and the introduction of skilled nurses; in fact the greatest help which the medical service of the army and navy can enjoy is that which comes from this volunteer and outside source. By the way, I wonder how many of you recall, or are familiar with, the beginnings of the Red Cross movement? So important has it become that its history should be well known to all. In June, 1859, was fought the bloody battle of Solferino, at the conclusion of which some 36,000 French, Sardinian and Austrian soldiers lay dead or dying on the field. The medical corps was, of course, absolutely inadequate to the work thrown upon them, and as usual thousands of wounded men had to care for themselves as best they could. A Swiss traveler, Henri Dunant, viewing the scenes, and being profoundly impressed by them, not only assisted in the work of relief, but wrote a book entitled, "A Souvenir of Solferino," in which he urged more humane, widespread and speedy aid to the wounded. M. Moynier, president of the Society of Public Utility, of Geneva, a man of independent means; Dr. Appia, a wise physician, and M. Ador, an eminent lawyer of Geneva, also became interested in the movement.

The attention of the General of the Swiss Army was called to it and his co-operation enlisted. In this way came about, in 1863, the formation of a permanent society for the relief of wounded soldiers. At a meeting held in October in the same year men from many countries joined in discussing the subject, and an international conference was held, which resulted in calling an international convention, to be held at Geneva in the autumn of 1864.

Such was the beginning of the Red Cross movement, which has now extended all over the world, and has afforded an opportunity for all races, creeds and nationalities to care for those who are made victims of war or pestilence, or who suffer from any other great disaster with which private charity is unable to cope. It marks a step in the evolution of mankind, and has now achieved such universal recognition that national governments and individual potentates are glad to join hands in the great work. A more concrete application of the same idea has been the comparatively recent formation of ambulance corps and later of nursing bureaus, within our own service, and the employment of trained nurses.

THE EVIL EYE

This has not been in all respects an easy matter to bring about, nevertheless it has redounded to the credit and to the welfare of all concerned. Never at any time were the sick and injured, either in private or in military practice, so well cared for as now, and America should lead the world today, as ever, in the adequacy of its provisions and the perfection of its methods. In private this is notably the case in ordinary hospital work, as seen by all travelers, upon the continent and in Great Britain, who take pains to make comparisons with the way in which things are done there and in our own country. Although Florence Nightingale immortalized herself by showing what woman could do on the battle field and in military camps, it has remained for Americans to improve upon the lessons which she taught, while at the same time revering her for her wonderful devotion to her self-imposed duty and her enthusiasm. In its performance the lessons of the Crimean and the Civil War, for instance, have left their impressions upon history in such a way as may never be erased, and certainly no one was ever more entitled to the designation of "angel of the sick room" than was Miss Nightingale.

Wars of conquest bring about curious results and in unexpected ways. While greed, lust and fanaticism have been the three great impelling and underlying motives for most of the wars which man thrusts upon his fellow-men, one far nobler motive has been the occasional and the only just cause of strife, namely, the desire for liberty; still this is always secondary and the product of some other man's or people's greed. As only by the cataclysms of the natural world has it been prepared for man's habitation, so by some wars have come benefits unforeseen, with an amelioration of the condition of mankind in general, which could not have been secured by any less drastic measures. It is, however, a sad commentary on man's intelligence that most honor is paid to those who have taken the most lives rather than to those who have saved them. No school boy in the remotest districts but is brought up with some trifling knowledge of the world's heroes, so-called, though they were In reality the world's wholesale murderers. Yet you may find many persons, credited with higher education, who are still densely ignorant of the benefits conferred by those two greatest discoveries in the world's history (both of Anglo-Saxon origin), anesthesia and antisepsis, who will talk entertainingly and at length of Darius, Caesar, Hannibal and the more modern military lights, yet who never heard of Morton nor of Lister. Yet if today you inquire what is doing in the various parliaments of the world you learn that the talk is ever of more numerous and more powerful engines of destruction, and that those in power have no time to devote to improvements in the army or navy medical service, and that it is even now impossible to secure anything like adequate attention to our needs in this direction.

Means of taking human life must be constantly at hand; means of saving it are of small importance until the emergency has arisen; and then the blame for inadequate provision of both means and men falls not where it belongs, on the politicians who would not look ahead, but upon the administration of the medical department, who work to the point of desperation and despair in times of peace, who keep perpetual vigil, with scant recognition of the sacredness of their purpose, and scant aid in its accomplishment. Are the lessons of the South African, the Spanish-American and the Russo-Japanese wars to be forgotten almost before they have been recited? Are we prepared today to give adequate care and attention to our soldiers and sailors were war in sight? You well know that we are not; every military or naval surgeon knows we are not; the medical profession generally knows it; and our legislators have been told it until we are tired of repeating it. Yet, what is the result? The same indifference on their part, the same ignorance of what it all means; and on the part of the public the same blindness and fatuous confidence that "everything is all right."

For instance, if an adequate medical service is to be built up for war there should be one officer to every 100 of enlisted men. Estimating that an army of at least 400,000 men would be required were we engaged with a first-class power- and what other would dare to engage with us?- this means 4,000 army surgeons. Of these at least one-fourth should be regular and experienced medical officers. In other words, there should be for such an army at least 1,000 medical officers in the regular service, and also at least 3,000 volunteer surgeons, professionally and physically equipped for such work. Should anyone object that this exceeds all the provisions of time past, the reply is ready and all sufficient, namely, that in time past all such provisions have been utterly inadequate; that the conditions of modern warfare have undergone an entire change, that a sick, wounded or disabled man is an encumbrance, and that it behooves us to prevent sickness, and to cure the disabled man as quickly as possible. Furthermore, advances in medicine and surgery have been so great that far more is now expected of the medical corps than ever before, and it is a duty which we owe to those who incur the dangers of fighting for us that we should care for them. We are, therefore, under the very highest moral obligation to give them our best, and enough of it. It must be a small inducement that we offer to men to fight our battles if we permit them to feel that they are not objects of our solicitude when sick or wounded.

There is another feature which we cannot disregard. So long as army regulations require that a man educated in advanced science spend much of his valuable time in acting as bookkeeper or clerk, there will be less inducement to enter the service, and it will consequently not attract men of highest proficiency. That which is required of you is complicated and exacting. You must be good bookkeepers, good sanitarians, and equally good surgeons, physicians and even obstetricians. Above all, you are expected to be able to keep all the men under your supervision ready for the "firing line" at a moment's notice. You have received the highest compliment which the State can pay when you have been adjudged versatile and competent enough to fill all these roles and do all these things. Moreover, as you gain promotion other things will be expected of you, even, I hope, the filling of the chairs in this modern Military Medical School. It is in a way the West Point of the medical corps, and it would seem as though there should not be the slightest difficulty in replenishing vacancies in its faculty by detail from your ranks. The collections and the literary labors of your corps constitute today treasures exceeded in value by but few if any in this, the Nation's Capital. The library, the museum and the archives of the medical department have been models from which all the nations of the earth have copied.

In this connection there occurs to me, by way of contrast, the story of a French surgeon's experiences when he undertook to teach anatomy in a conquered and reconstructed country. After the French occupation of Egypt, Mehemet Ali took it into his head to introduce European civilization into Africa, and imported all sorts of artists, scientists and medical men, among them a practitioner of Marseilles, a true Bohemian in the modern acceptance of the expression, who presented himself in most seedy apparel, saying, "I am a doctor of medicine, with plenty of courage, but no clothes; I want to try my fortune." This man was Dr. Clot, who rapidly became a favorite of the Viceroy. He soon learned Arabic so as to speak it fluently, and in six months not only received an army commission, and became a Bey, but took the chair of anatomy in the newly organized school of medicine. Conditions were all against him. Mussulman fanaticism and the prohibitions of the Koran opposed all anatomical pursuits, and so soon as he proposed a dissection there was a general explosion. By Mohammedan ceremonial one who even touches a dead body is thereby rendered "unclean" for seven days. The Ulemas, the Muftis, and all of the other fanatics, demanded of the Viceroy the closure of the school, and declared dissection a sacrilegious profanation.

Mehemet refused this, and ordered Clot Bey to commence his demonstrations. Then one day happened the following incident: The professor, scalpel In hand, standing alongside the cadaver, began to open the thorax, when one of the students, either from sheer fanaticism, or more bold than the others, jumped upon him and stabbed him with a poignard. The blade slid over the ribs, and Clot Bey, perceiving that he was not seriously hurt, applied a piece of plaster to the wound, observing as he did so, "We were speaking of the disposition of the sternum and the ribs, and I now can Illustrate to you why a blow directed from above has so little chance of penetrating the cavity of the thorax." He continued his lectures, and turned out some skillful practitioners. He became an officer of almost every order in the world, and acquired more than sixty decorations, although he never wore but one, the red rosette of his own country. (Med. Times and Gazette, September 19, 1868.)

While just such an experience may never be duplicated again, the Philippines, or some other country yet to fall under our rule, may afford an opportunity for a similar display of *sang froid*.

While no one may see far into the future, the maxim, "In time of peace prepare for war," is as true of the medical department as of any. Were it a state secret no one would breathe it here, but it is lamentably true and publicly known that even now we are not prepared as we should be. The awful lessons of the Spanish War have been forgotten. West Point officers have until comparatively recently received no instruction in camp sanitation. Some of us worked hard a while ago to have at least elementary instruction in it introduced into their curriculum. As an illustration I believe that today they are taught more about horse's feet and how to keep them in good condition, than about those of their men. Line officers, especially volunteer, have never been too ready to locate their camps where water and drainage were the best, and the awful mortality of the Spanish War was mainly due to preventable disease, while this was due to stupid and inexcusable disregard, on the part of officers of the line (mainly volunteer) of the advice of their medical officers.

But, after all, gentlemen, the discouragements you will

meet with will be far fewer than those with which your predecessors had to contend, while the pleasant side of your lives will be far pleasanter than was theirs. In fact, I think your lives have in many respects fallen in pleasanter places than have ours. Discipline and order protect you to a large extent from quackery and idiocy. The fads of the day disappear before the appearance of the flag and the sound of the drum. So-called Christian Science finds no place in your curriculum, and it will be long, I trust, before the army chaplain tinctures the military hospital with sectarian therapeutics or an Emanuel church cult. If by entering the army one may escape disgusting influences of this character, then it may become such a refuge that it shall thereby be made both inviting and invincible.

It is pleasing to those of us who cooperated in the movement, to have the assurances of the Surgeon General that the establishment of the Medical Reserve Corps has been of actual benefit to the regular Army Medical Department. While the military rank to which its members found themselves suddenly elevated was not so lofty as to cause any attacks of vertigo, none having been up to the present day reported, it at least gives us satisfaction to realize that help may thus be afforded from private life, and that a closer rapport has been effected. And now it is well nigh as difficult a task to appropriately conclude these remarks as to begin them.

Men come and go; a few leave imprints of their footsteps; the vast majority make no impression that lingers. "Some when they die, die all; their moldering clay Is but an emblem of their memories; The space quite closes up through which they passed." Fain would I believe that many of you would make enduring records. Yet each can do his best, and I doubt not each will do it. You have so much to encourage you, so comparatively little to hamper or hold back. Glorious is your work, glorious may be your fulfillment of it. We have lived in a goodly time; you will enjoy one still more goodly. With scientific progress, whose like the world has never known, and with an altruism which makes the world constantly better, you will be able to do things never done by your predecessors.

"Tis coming up the steeps of time.
And this old world is growing brighter!
We may not sec its dawn sublime.
Yet high hopes make the heart throb lighter!
Our dust may slumber underground
When it awakens the world in wonder;
But we have felt it gathering 'round!
We have heard its voice of distant thunder.
'Tis coming! Yes, 'tis coming!

'Tis coming now, that glorious time
Foretold by seers and sung in story.
For which, when thinking was a crime.
Souls leaped to heaven from scaffolds gory!
They passed. But lo ! the work they wrought!
Now the crowned hopes of centuries blossom,
The lightning of their living thought
Is flashing through us, brain and bosom;
'Tis coming! Yes, 'tis coming."

XI: THE EVOLUTION OF THE SURGEON FROM THE BARBER

If one attempt to scan the field of the history of medicine, to take note of all the fallacies and superstitions which have befogged men's minds, and brought about what now seem to be the most absurd and revolting views and practices of times gone by, and if one search deliberately for that which is of curious nature, or calculated to serve as a riddle difficult of solution, he will scarcely in the tomes which he may consult find anything stranger than the close connection, nay, even the identity maintained for centuries, between the trade of the barber and the craft of the surgeon. Even after having studied history and the various laws passed at different times, he will still miss the predominant yet concealed reason for this state of affairs. This will be found to be, in the words of Paget, the "maintenance of vested rights as if they were better than the promotion of knowledge." He will wonder also why women were licensed to practice surgery in the fourteenth century and prevented in the nineteenth, or why specialties were legally recognized in the sixteenth century only to lose their dignity and identity a little later.

In thus attempting to consider the relations which have existed in time past between barbers and surgeons I must ask you to remember that there was a time when bleeding was deemed necessary for the cure of almost all ailments, and that after the Church had condemned the shedding of blood by any of her officials it was most natural to turn for assistance to the barbers, who were supposed to be dexterous with sharp instruments, with basins and with towels. Thus it happened that when the barbers found themselves permitted to perform this sole act they naturally ventured further and practiced many parts of minor surgery independently of the ecclesiastics. Moreover there persist today in Europe many relics of the old customs, and the barber surgeon is still a common figure in Germany, and particularly in Russia, where the really educated surgeons are still too few for a vast and widespread population. It must be remembered also that the Church gradually imbued men's minds with a horror of a dead body, and of the profanation which followed having anything to do with it, and surrounded the study of anatomy with every possible obstacle and obloquy; even to such an extent that to be known as having dissected a human body was to be exposed to indignity, assault and even death. It was, therefore only intense yearning for knowledge, on the part of earnest men, which then permitted anatomical instruction to be given or encouraged.

During the middle ages the greatest medical school in the world was situated at Salernum (or Salerno), but a short distance from Naples. This is not the place in which to discuss its history, although it became famous above almost every other institution of learning of any kind, and though, by one of the freaks of history, even the site of the buildings is now lost and no one seems to know just where they stood. In his time, namely, in 1240, the Emperor Frederick II was the great patron of this college; his decrees concerning the regulation of the study and practice of medicine deserve attention today. A part of one of his enactments reads as follows:

"Since it is possible for a man to understand medical science only if he has previously learned something of logic, we ordain that no one shall be permitted to study medicine until he has given his attention to logic for three years. After these three years he may if he wishes proceed to the study of medicine." And again: "No surgeon shall be allowed to practice until he has submitted certificates in writing, of the teachers of the faculty of medicine, that he has spent at least one year in that part of medical science which gives skill in the practice of surgery, that in the college he has diligently and especially studied the anatomy of the human body, and is also thoroughly experienced in the way in which operations are successfully performed and healing afterwards brought about."

THE EVIL EYE

When first we hear of medical men in Great Britain they were commonly spoken of as leeches, as among the Danes and Saxons; later the clergy introduced books from Rome, and almost every Monastery had some brother possessed of more or less knowledge of the medicine of the day. The College of Salernum later gave great impetus to the study of medicine, even before the days of William the Conqueror, which was strengthened by the influence emanating from Naples, and particularly from Montpellier. For centuries the Catholic clergy were almost the only persons with sufficient education to study and practice physic; which profession became in time so lucrative that many of the monks abandoned their monasteries, neglecting their religious duties, and applied themselves to the study of medicine.

To such an extent was this true that in 1163 the Council of Tours forbade monks staying out of the monastery for more than two months at a time, or teaching or practicing physic. In taking this action the Council only repeated what had been ordained by decree of Henry III in 1216, and by the second Council of Lateran in 1139. No restraint was at first placed upon the secular clergy, and many of the Bishops and other church dignitaries gained both money and honor by acting as physicians to Kings and Princesses. Next to the clergy the Jews possessed the largest share of learning. Their nomadic life permitted an intercourse with the different nations of the world, which was denied to most others, and there were many who studied medicine and practiced, not only among those of their own race but among Moors and Christians alike. The priests became extremely jealous of Jewish physicians and of lay surgeons, and endeavored to secure through Rome a formal excommunication of all who committed themselves to the care of a Jew, while by canon law no Jew might give medicine to a Christian. But so celebrated were the Jewish physicians, and so superior to everything else was men's desire for life and strength, that even the power of Rome could not exclude them from practice. Still less could the clergy restrain the lay surgeons from the performance of their craft, and though it would appear that at first, in England, the priests were not disposed to separate surgery from medicine, the Pope became jealous of so much interruption to the duties of the clergy and looked upon the manual part of surgery as detracting from clerical dignity.

Accordingly were made numerous attempts to debar priests from the performance of surgical operations. In 1215 the ecclesiastics were prohibited by Pope Innocent III from undertaking any operation involving the shedding of blood, while by Boniface VIII at the close of the thirteenth century, and Clement V, about the beginning of the fourteenth century, surgery was formally separated from physic and the priests positively forbidden to practice it. It is to the Church then that we owe this absolute abandonment of surgery to an illiterate and grasping laity. For some time, however, the priests kept their hold upon surgery by instructing their servants, the barbers, who were employed to shave their own priestly beards, in the performance of minor operations. It was these men, who were in some degree qualified by the instruction of the clergy, who first assumed the title of barber surgeons, and who gradually formed a great fraternity. In France it was in the reign of Louis XIV that the hairdressers were formally separated from the barber-surgeons, the latter being incorporated as a distinct medical body. In London it was in 1375 that the Company of Barbers were practically divided into two sections, containing respectively those who practiced shaving, and those who practiced surgery.

In 1460 the surgeons were finally incorporated by themselves as the Guild of Surgeons and took their place as one of the liveried companies of the city of London. Similar separation occurred in the original great Guild of Weavers, who divided into the Woolen Drapers and Linen Armorers, the latter afterwards becoming the wealthy and powerful Company of Merchant Tailors. To trace the history of the London Company of Barbers a little more fully, it was first formed in 1308 and incorporated in 1462 by a charter. In one of the statutes of Henry

VIII it was enacted that: "No person using any shaving or barbery in London shall occult (i. e. practice) any surgery, letting of blood or other matter except only drawing of teeth."

In 1540 Parliament passed an act allowing the United Companies of Barbers and Surgeons each to have yearly the bodies of four criminals for dissection. In 15 1 8 the barbers and surgeons were united in one company; the former being restricted from all operations except tooth drawing, and the latter having to abandon shaving and hair dressing. It is interesting also to note that in Oxford, for instance, the Barbers, Surgeons, Waferers and Makers of "Singing bread" were all of the same fellowship, from 1348 to 1500; when, at last, the Cappers, or knitters of caps, were united to them, in 1551, the barbers and waferers abrogated their charter and took one in the name of the city, until 1675, when they received a charter from the University. The London Guild of Surgeons appears to have been first a mere fraternity which had incorporated itself, and to have originated from an association of the military barber surgeons who had been trained in the hundred years war with France, 1337 to 1444. Its membership, however, was select, and when the physicians declined an alliance with it, it amalgamated with the barber companies in 1540. The United Company of Barbers and Surgeons was peculiar in that strangers and those who were not free men were admitted, while the journeymen of the craft formed a subordinate body within the company.

In 1745 the surgeons separated from the barbers and formed a surgeon's company which rapidly acquired influence. By a foolish blunder it forfeited its charter in 1496 but was subsequently incorporated by George III, in 1800, as the Royal College of Surgeons in London; a body which has since maintained its identity, grown tremendously in wealth and strength, and having become one of the licensing bodies of England, has acquired the finest collection of books and specimens in the world and has numbered the brightest intellects which the English surgical profession has contained. In Dublin the Barber Surgeons were incorporated as a guild by charter granted by Henry VI, in 1446. In 1576 they were amalgamated with the independent surgeons, and by Queen Elizabeth with the barber surgeons and wig-makers. This confraternity was dissolved in 1784 and the College of Surgeons founded immediately afterwards. In Edinburgh the barbers and surgeons were united in 1505, to be separated at about the same time as elsewhere in Great Britain.

During the eighteenth and nineteenth centuries on the continent medicine and surgery were abruptly separated, and the latter was almost entirely in the hands of the barbers. For hundreds of years the dissection of corpses and the embalming of those who could afford it, were in the hands of first the butchers and later of the barbers. The greatest contempt was everywhere shown for one who attempted any surgery. If for instance a nobleman while being bled by a barber received the slightest harm the poor barber was heavily fined, while, should the gentleman die, the culprit was given into the hands of the dead man's relatives to be dealt with as they desired. Throughout the monasteries and whenever the influence of the Church was felt it was forbidden to the monks, who had the monopoly of knowledge, to perform any surgical operation since the Church abhorred the shedding of blood. (I leave it to defenders of the Faith to reconcile this abhorrence with the persecutions of heretics and the tortures of the Inquisition permitted by the same Church.)

For hundreds of years the monks were not allowed to wear a beard; this necessitated the employment of tonsors ("tonsorial-artists" they call themselves today) to whom was left also the performance of anything that partook of the nature of an operation, such as bleeding, bandaging, etc. This calling, was however, recognized as a most inferior one, and the barbers, like the bathkeeper, the shepherd and the hangman, were not considered of good repute. Consequently, such an one was not eligible for membership in any other guilds or fraternities. In

THE EVIL EYE

1406 the Emperor Wenzel was rescued from prison, in Prague, by the daughter of a bathkeeper; in gratitude he made her his mistress, and declared both barbers and bathkeepers to be respectable; but having lost his position his decree had no weight, and not until 1548, in Augsburg, were they really made eligible to the guilds. At this time their most dignified labor was the sharpening of instruments. In 1696 Leopold I decreed their profession to be an art, and gave it a position above that of the apothecary so that in their most dignified occupation they were elevated to the making of ointments and plasters.

As surgery has for the profession of barber surgery to thank the existence upon man of a beard, so the European continent may thank the Crusaders of the eleventh century for having necessitated the existence of the bathkeeper, because of the leprosy which they brought home from the East. During the Crusades, as is well known, there were founded numerous Orders having for their original purpose the care and protection of pilgrims and injured soldiers. The three most celebrated Orders were the Knights of St. John, the Knights Templar and the Teutonic Order. Were this the place it would be most interesting to go Into a history of these religio-medico military orders, and show how from most devout purposes and humble origin they grew Into despotic and tyrannical associations of great power, which It finally took all the force of Church and State to suppress. As the then humble and enthusiastic members of these Orders returned from the Holy Land they established hospitals for the care of lepers, who became very numerous in Europe. For instance it is stated that in France, in 1225, there were two thousand hospitals for this purpose, while the King Louis the Great founded, In 1260, a special hospital for those made blind by Egyptian ophthalmia. It is well known also that during the middle ages there was the greatest neglect of the ordinary canons of cleanliness both among the upper and lower classes. The number of hospitals and cloisters dedicated to the lepers being insufficient, bath houses were built and bathkeepers were engaged in order, so far as possible, to prevent the spread of leprosy. At this time the bathkeeper was permitted to bathe and cup, later also to bleed, although the bleeding was required to be done in the bathkeepers' own house, since he was not usually permitted to enter a patient's house. As bathing became less necessary for purposes already mentioned the bathkeeper took to imitating the barber, though much later, and not until about 1750 in some countries, were they permitted to do this publicly, and only after having passed the examinations to which the barber was also subjected. In Prussia they were only allowed to treat wounds and chronic diseases, and so It came about that by the beginning of the eighteenth century a really conscientious and efficient barber surgeon was supposed to have served an apprenticeship In large hospitals, to have witnessed the work of noted surgeons and to have served in the Army or Navy. He was also supposed to be something of a linguist and to know a little botany; particularly was he expected to be conversant with anatomy, although there was a sad lack of cadavers- which was atoned for by the use of carcasses of animals, for the main part swine.

Eckardt, writing at this time of the sixteen different virtues of a barber, enumerated, first of all, fear of God; then that he should be careful, prudent, temperate, and ready to use both hands with equal dexterity; he claimed that "Arrogance seems most prevalent among barbers, as a common saying would imply 'barbers are proud animals.'" He expressed his surprise also at the envy and malice between bathkeepers and barbers, and advised them both to consult physicians and other masters.

The customs of the time must be blamed for this lamentable condition of affairs. The boy who was destined to become a barber was apprenticed at a time when he had scarcely learned to write. If he could write legibly and read a little Latin no one dared refuse him. He learned to shave and went from house to house for this purpose, spending the little time remaining in sharpening knives, spreading plasters, picking lint, taking care of children, doing all menial duties, and using the same light as the housemaid because it would have been disrespectful to his master's wife to use any other. After years of this work he was gradually taken to visit patients and then was taught how to bleed, cup, apply leeches, extract teeth and administer clysters. His master knowing nothing of anatomy could give him no instruction, though by the laws of apprenticeship he was bound to do so. Before concluding this apprenticeship he was supposed to pass an examination, which his master's laziness usually permitted him to escape. He then presented the master with some silver instruments and was dismissed with an injunction to be thankful that such a miserable specimen of God's creatures had ever been taught to shave a beard or spread a plaster. He now became a journeyman, still living at the house of his master, and was not allowed to marry; after a while he received a paltry sum as wages, got his dinners free and began to dabble on his own account. Study was out of the question; these men could not understand what little they did read and served the community mainly as bearers of tales. After some years of activity as journeyman they could become masters by applying to the authorities, presenting certificates, and passing an examination before the physicians of the district.

Prussia was the first country to appreciate the necessity of regulating medical practice, and the barbers and bathkeepers were placed under the control of the Medical College founded, in 1685, by Prince Frederick William. In 1724 this institution attained its greatest activity, having a subordinate school in each province. In 1725 King Frederick William issued a famous edict which did much to regulate medical affairs throughout the kingdom, and directed among other things that barbers and bathkeepers should "lead a religious, temperate, retired and sober life, in order to be at their best whenever their services were required." When their business was not sufficiently good they assumed other cares, as, for instance, one man was surgeon, municipal judge and post-master all at once. They were extremely envious of each other and often dabbled in medicine without permission. It was not until 1779 that the bathkeepers were permitted to rank in Prussia with the barbers, and were allowed to use more than four basins, the bathkeepers' guild being incorporated with that of the barber.

There being no temptation to enter these ranks it is not strange that so late even as 1790 good surgeons were rare in Germany; not one in fifty of the barbers really knowing the first principles of the work they were supposed to perform. It came to such a pass that surgeons were compelled to shave and perform other duties of the hairdresser, for no surgeon, however skilled, was allowed to practice as such, unless he was the proprietor of a head-shaving and bathing establishment, with assistants and apprentices, and belonged to the barbers' guild, or unless he was favored by Royal exemption. It was the general lament in Germany, all through the 18th century, that German surgeons were educated in barber shops. Even by the middle of that century the practice of surgery was not considered an honorable business, and those who practiced it were not permitted to carry a sword, neither was a surgeon admitted into society nor tolerated among physicians; moreover when unsuccessful he was bitterly and relentlessly pursued. Under existing conditions the Reichstag either could or would do nothing to alleviate the distressing condition. The physician boasted of his education and treated the surgeon and his craft with disdain, holding that surgery sustained the same relation to medicine that geometry does to higher mathematics and physics. All this time, however, while the physician contented himself with disdaining surgeons he made no attempt to elevate the craft nor to himself study and adorn it. Even by the beginning of the nineteenth century there were scarcely any physicians In Europe who could diagnose a surgical case, while dentistry they claimed called for no more skill than that sufficient for tooth extraction. It was even claimed that so long as the people generally were neglectful of their teeth the physician, or even the surgeon, should be ashamed to concern himself with dentistry. Von Siebold, in his day, deplored the position of the surgeon; his large military experience had shown him the difficulties with which he had to contend before he could enter society, while his ambitions and high motives were scorned. Even the peasantry were bitterly opposed to all operations. So intense were their feelings that he repeatedly removed his patients to other towns before performing operations.

Nevertheless it was true that there were the best of reasons for lack of confidence in any barber who dropped his razor for the purpose of treating a fracture, a hernia or an obstetric case. The State required a barber surgeon to call in a physician in all complicated surgical cases. In such a case the physician demanded the control of the case and reserved to himself the right to judge of what was required. He would not even consider a surgeon who had obtained the doctorate as his equal. Such consultations resulted in little but quarrels and disagreeable scenes. If a village contained no physician the surgeon treated also internal diseases, though he was not allowed to use strong medicines. Every district had its special surgeon who, alone, had charge of several villages where he had the right to keep journeymen and apprentices and to do shaving and cupping. In the Prussian capital city only twenty German and six French surgeons were allowed to practice in 1725, besides the court and private surgeons.

Until 1808 every German surgeon carried on a medico-legal business which was later separated from his surgery. In 1782 there were three classes of surgeons; from the lower one might be promoted to a higher after an examination. In Austria, in 1805, there were doctors of surgery who were required to show a general knowledge of medicine and who had the same rights as the physicians; there were also medical surgeons who could practice under restrictions, and bathkeepers for minor surgery. After the year 1773 barbers and bathkeepers were both spoken of in Austria as surgeons; this was to break up the disputes between them. According to an official fee-bill holding good in Prussia in 1815, the highest fee that could be charged for an operation was for lithotomy in adults, the maximum limit being about M. 140 ($35), while the majority of operations ranged from M. 20 to M. 50 ($5.00 to $13.00 expressed in U. S. money). Of course this was at a time when the value of money was much greater than now.

As already made plain, it was the Church which by its decrees brought about the separation of surgery from medicine, a condition not existing during the palmy days of Greece and Rome. Even the University of Paris at one time refused to admit a student who had not forsworn the study of surgery, while the denouncement of anatomy and surgery alike was promulgated by both papal bulls and clerical decrees. While many of the physicians considered surgery too burdensome a study, and many others had a severe prejudice against it, the principal cause operating to keep them apart was probably the fact that for surgeons there was absolutely no social position. In 1774 Mederer was made Professor of Surgery in Freiburg, in Breisgau; he delivered his opening address on the wisdom and necessity of combining medicine and surgery. As a result he was persecuted by the public, insulted by students, abused by surgeons and constantly threatened with personal assault. He maintained his position, however, and fought against the prejudice. Twenty two years later, when he left Freiburg, he referred in his last lecture to his early experience. By this time public opinion had been so changed that the students serenaded him and humbly apologized for what their predecessors had done.

Mederer could then see the success of his efforts in that the constitution of France contained a clause combining medicine and surgery, and the Royal Sanitary Commissioners of Vienna had unanimously resolved in favor of such union. The movement begun by Mederer was continued by men like Richter, Von Siebold, Loder and others. In 1797, or over a hundred years ago, the Electoral Academy of Erfurt offered a prize for the best essay on the subject "Is it necessary and possible to combine medicine and surgery theoretically as well as practically?"

Fourteen papers were submitted, of which twelve were in favor of union. Nevertheless the Academy awarded the prize to the only writer who had opposed such union. His reasons for such opposition were most puerile, as were all the arguments subsequently advanced against it. Nevertheless a great step was taken in advance, when the guilds and fraternities of barbers and bathkeepers were abolished, in which good work Vienna, in 1783, took the lead. It was then declared that shaving was the business of the hair-dresser, and that barber surgeons must attend lectures in surgery and anatomy. Bavaria followed in 1804, and four years later, in Prussia, no one was permitted to practice surgery without having studied medicine. The rules of 1786 regulating the respective positions and duties between physicians and surgeons were annulled in 1808, and by 1811 the barber license was no longer essential for the practice of surgery, the privileges of the barber, as such, being abolished, while for his trade only a common license was needed.

XII: THE STORY OF THE DISCOVERY OF THE CIRCULATION

A Study of the Times and Labors of William Harvey

Address delivered at the Annual Commencement of the Medical Department of the University of Chicago, (Rush Medical College), June 13, 1906.

History in general is but a record of the succession of great events or epochs which have molded the world's affairs. That which is of the greatest import in the life of the individual may count for little in the lives of his contemporaries, and yet it must be said that in the events of today there has occurred a great epoch in the life of each of you, presumably the most important as yet in your personal records. This day is then in your personal histories one of the greatest importance. It is desirable, therefore, that your lives be so molded and influenced by it that you may long hence look back to it and recall its significance. I do not know what advice I can give you which will be more fruitful of results, than that among your studies you include that of the lives of the great men who have molded destiny and made the world's history. Their lives were modified by little things, as have been and will be yours, and yet out of small matters grew for them and for us some of the most far reaching effects. Select the really great men of whom you best happen to know and analyze their characters that you may appreciate how they have become great; while if they have, as all great men have, traits of smallness, study even wherein they are small, and how such faults may be avoided.

History runs as does a fairly steady stream, save that every now and then some event abruptly diverts its course or influences its current. It has been so, for instance, with the history of medicine. For the first sixteen hundred years of the

THE EVIL EYE

Christian era men engaged in the crude practices of our profession, utterly ignorant of the course of the blood, as well as of its purposes. Then appeared upon the scene a man who did his own thinking, who was willing to free himself from the shackles of the past, to observe nature and to reason therefrom. In this way came suddenly upon the world, as it were, an appreciation of the Circulation of the Blood, than which perhaps no event in medical history has been of greater importance or reflected more credit upon its demonstrator. It is my purpose, then, today to try to tell you, in a semipopular way, how William Harvey came to make this great discovery, as well as to give you some idea of the difficulties under which he worked, and of the men and influences that surrounded him, believing that rather than spend a half hour in humorous platitudes which may provoke a smile, but which are quickly forgotten, It Is much better to try to implant something which may linger a while in your memories, and sufficiently Impress you with the value of observation and inductive reasoning, since if you become thus fully impressed you will be spared in the future many sad errors of speech and even of thought.

Before telling the story of Harvey's life and work let us study for a few moments the general condition of affairs in Europe, in order that we may better understand the men whose influence surrounded him, as well as the spirit of the times and men's habits of thought. Among the monarchs reigning in various parts of Europe during Harvey's time there were, for instance. In that part of the Empire of the West which was called Germany, Rudolph II, Matthias and Ferdinand. In Sweden reigned King Sigismund, Charles IX, the great monarch Gustavus Adolphus, and Queen Christine. In Prussia the throne had been occupied by Joachim, George William and Frederick William, as electors, this being before the days of the Prussian kings. In Russia the Czars Boris Godunow, Michael Theodore and Alexis had occupied the throne.

France had but recently passed through the inhuman

butchery of the massacre of St. Bartholomew and its accompanying persecution of the Huguenots, under Charles IX, who expressed the hope that not a single Huguenot would be left alive to reproach him with the deed, but who died himself soon after the massacre, which is said to have caused him bitter remorse. Charles had been succeeded by his brother Henry III, a weak, fickle and vicious monarch, whose weakness caused him to be embroiled in civil strife, which was only concluded by his own assassination at the hands of a Dominican friar. Then came Henry IV, he of Navarre, afterwards surnamed The Great, who fought the famous battle of Ivry in 1590, and who reigned for twenty-one years, the greatest and most popular sovereign who ever occupied the throne of France. Notwithstanding his noble qualities he did not succeed in preserving his court from many of the contaminations of the age, and in his reign it is said that no less than 4,000 French gentlemen were killed in duels, chiefly arising out of quarrels about women. He was succeeded by Louis XIII, who was still on the throne when Harvey died.

In Harvey's own country James I was occupying the throne when Harvey appeared upon the scene. He was that royal pedant whom the Duke of Sully pronounced "the wisest fool in Europe." After his death, and when Charles I ascended the throne during his twenty-fifth year, in 1625, Harvey was preparing to publish his great work. It was this Charles I who retained as a favorite the worthless scoundrel Buckingham, whose misconduct in Spain prevented the proposed marriage of the king with the Spanish Infanta and brought about the Civil War. It was because of the cost of this war, and of the king's disputes with Parliament regarding the matter, that England was rent between the conflicts of the Cavaliers and the Roundheads, two of the consequences of this intestine strife being the execution of the Earl of Strafford and of Archbishop Laud. The troubles thus engendered finally cost the life of the king himself, who was beheaded In 1649. Harvey even lived to see the first half of the short tenure of office of Cromwell as the Great Protector, and was perhaps fortunate in dying before began the reign of that odious profligate Charles II.

It is worth while to inquire for a moment what was doing on this side of the ocean at this period which we have now under consideration. In 1607 Virginia was settled by the English, in 1614 New York, by the Dutch, in 1620 Massachusetts and, three years later, New Hampshire, by the English Puritans; In 1624 New Jersey, by the Dutch, in 1627 Delaware by Swedes and Finns, in 1630 Maine, by the English, in 1634 Maryland, by Irish Catholics, in 1635 Connecticut, by English Puritans. Thus it will be seen that the active period of Harvey's life was synchronous with the beginnings of our colonial activities. Very little knowledge of what was going on in the then world of science was brought to this country at this period of its existence, however, and it was many years before in these colonies there were any exhibitions of scientific interest save in extremely scattered and sporadic cases.

Among Harvey's literary associates were a number of celebrated English poets, for example- Marlowe (1593), J Spenser (1598), Beaumont (1615), Shakespeare (1615), Herbert (1635), Ben Jonson (1637), Massinger (1639). Lord Bacon died a year or two after the appearance of Harvey's book, while Baron Napier, the inventor of logarithms, had passed away. His contemporaries in Italy, where he had studied, included Tasso (1595) and Galileo (1645). Rubens had died in 1640, Michael Angelo in 1564 and Titian in 1576. In France, Calvin, the practical murderer of Servetus, had passed away in 1564, Beza died in 1605, Descartes in 1650, Pascal in 1662 and Gassendi in 1655. Portugal had produced but one great figure in the 16th century, namely Camoens, who died in 1579. In Spain, Loyola, the ascetic and fanatic founder of the Jesuits, had joined the great majority in 1556; but Cervantes did not die until 1616, Lope de Vega in 1635, Velasquez in 1660 and Calderon in 1667.

In Germany some great figures had but recently disappeared. Paracelsus died in 1541, Copernicus in 1543,

Luther in 1546, Hans Holbein in 1554, and Melancthon in 1560. Mercator, who introduced a new method of cartography, died in 1594, Tycho Brahe in 1601, Keppler in 1631, Van Dyck in 1641, Grotlus, the great scholar, in 1645, Rembrandt In 1668 and Spinoza in 1677.

In philosophy, skepticism was the prevailing doctrine in the time of Harvey. It had been founded a hundred years previously by Montaigne, and continued by Charron, the chaplain of Queen Margaret of Navarre, who died in 1603, and who declared all religion to be opposed to human reason- a remarkable attitude for a chaplain to assume. Opposed to the skepticism of Harvey's day was the mystic, Cabalistic or supernatural philosophy especially represented by Bohme, a peasant shoemaker, uneducated and yet wonderfully gifted. He had been the philosophical colleague of that great Meistersinger, Hans Sachs. Later philosophers and thinkers, yet belonging to Harvey's time, were Pascal, the great Jansenist, who discovered the variations of atmospheric pressure at different levels, and Malebranche, who figures prominently in the history of philosophy.

Descartes, who died in 1650, held the pineal gland to be the seat of the soul. He was the discoverer of the laws of refraction of light and furnished the explanation for the rainbow. He attained greatest eminence in mathematics, physics and philosophy, and was one of the inventors of modern algebra. One of his greatest opponents was that noble Jew, Spinoza, whose colleagues had expelled him from the Sanhedrin to the sound of the trombone. The Italian Dominican Campanella, who died in 1639, considered the foundation of knowledge to be supernatural revelation and its perception by the senses. In spite of these views he came before The Inquisition on a charge of heresy and of cooperation with the Turks, was tortured by the rack, and imprisoned for thirty years.

The mystic or Cabalistic notions of Harvey's day have

just been mentioned. Under them we may recognize many degenerate products and amalgamations of the real doctrines of Paracelsus. The doctrines of the Rosicrucians, as well as of Zoroaster and the Cabala, were revived and made to do strange work. There was, for instance, that Sir Kenelm Digby, who died in 1605, a King's chamberlain, who posed among the English as a so-called Rosicrucian. It was he who suggested the famous "sympathetic powder" which was to be applied to the weapon by which a wound had been inflicted, after which the weapon was anointed and dressed two or three times a day, while the wound itself was carefully bound up with dressings and left alone for a week. This was perhaps much the better course, but it will show what strange notions prevailed in those days.

What it meant to run counter to ecclesiastical policy and theological dogma appears not only in such tragedies as terminated the lives of Bruno and many other martyrs to science, but in such facts as these; for instance, when in 1624, just when Harvey was preparing to publish his work, some young chemists in Paris, seeing the benefit of the experimental method, broke away from Aristotle and the canons of theological reasoning, the faculty of theology appealed to the Parliament of Paris, which latter prohibited all such researches, under the severest penalties. This was the time too when such exhibitions as the following were altogether too frequent- One Quaresimo, of Lodi, came out with a ponderous work entitled "A Historical, Theological and Moral Explanation of the Holy Land," in which he devoted great space to the question of The Dead Sea and the salt pillar supposed to represent Lot's wife, dividing a long chapter upon the subject into three parts, dealing with the method and the locality of this transformation and the question of the existence at that time of her saline remains. Thus, with his peculiar powers of reasoning, he was able to decide the exact point where the saline change took place, and finally showed that the statue was still in existence.

Lord Bacon was also an older contemporary of Harvey,

having been born in 1561 and dying in 1626, shortly after the appearance of Harvey's great work. His services to analytic science need no description here, but it is worth while to remember that Harvey, like many others, must have come under his influence and have profited by his teachings in logic and analysis. At about the time when Harvey made known his discovery Bacon was publishing his views of the laws of transmission and reflection of sound. Great man as he was, with a keen foresight into the value of the recent inventions of the compass, gun-powder and printing, he nevertheless was himself so narrow, in some respects, that he placed but little value upon the discovery of Copernicus. He, however, paved the way for one in some respects still greater, namely Isaac Newton, who, however, had scarcely attained man's stature when Harvey died.

How much we owe to the two great Bacons of history one cannot indicate in this short resume. Roger Bacon (1214-1292) seems to have been the first great thinker along truly scientific lines. He was more than a mere chemist while, as White says, more than three centuries before Francis Bacon advocated the experimental method Roger Bacon had practiced it, and in many directions. He did more than anyone else in the middle ages to direct thought into fruitful paths, and only now are we finding out how nearly he reached some of the principal doctrines of modern philosophy and chemistry. Most important of all, his methods were even greater than his results, and this at a time when "theological subtilizing" was the only passport to reputation for scholarship. It was Avicenna, the Arabian, who perhaps first announced substantially the modern theory of geology, accounting for changes in the earth's surface by suggesting a stone-making force, but the presence of fossils in the rocks had been always a thorn in the sides of the theologians. It was Leonardo da Vinci, that versatile genius in science and art, who, previous to Harvey's generation, suggested true notions as to the origin of fossils, while, in Harvey's time, Bernard Palissy, another artist, vehemently contended for their correctness. Still, even at Harvey's death, neither geology nor paleontology had come anywhere near scientific accuracy.

The Academia del Lyncei, so-called from its seal, which bore the image of a fox, was founded in Rome in 1603. In France The Academy of Science was not founded until 1665, in Germany The Society of Naturalists and Physicians in 1652, and the British Royal Society in 1665.

In matters of general interest it may be worth while to say that in architecture the general style of The Renaissance was changed for the more substantial Barocco, while the more formal and limited style of church music had given away to musical drama, i. e., opera, albeit in very crude form. The first newspaper had appeared at Antwerp in 1605, the first German paper being published in Frankfort in 1615, and The London Weekly News making its first appearance in 1620. Tobacco, which had been brought over by Raleigh in 1560, had come into quite general use, while coffee, tea and chocolate had gained in public esteem. When coffee was first introduced in England it sold for about $28 a pound. The first coffee house appears to have been established in Constantinople, in the middle of the 16th century, while the first coffee house in London was not opened until a century later.

The barbers still retained their ascendancy, and the bath keepers had scarcely lost their position next to the barbers. It was not until Harvey had reached a ripe age that the barbers were required in Germany to pass an examination, in which they had to prove not only their knowledge but the legitimacy of their birth, and the fact that they had studied for three years and had worked for three years more as apprentices. Anatomy was studied quite generally, sometimes upon human bodies. A dissecting room had been established in Dresden In 1617, in which stuffed bears, at that time a great rarity, were preserved with other curiosities. In 1623 Rolfink, at Jena, arranged for public dissection upon the bodies of all executed malefactors, delegates being present thereat from various other institutions. It is worth while to mention that in Frankfort, for instance, during the expiration of 65 years, but seven dissections were made, and that these were always accompanied by a celebration which lasted several days. Vienna did not possess a skeleton in 1668, and Strassburg did not have one until 1671. Yet it is of interest to remember that the anatomical plates, like those often published today, which are meant to be lifted off in layers, existed even at this period. On the other hand, botanical gardens and chemical laboratories existed in several of the universities- in Strassburg, for instance.

In 1619- in Oxford in 1622. Fabricius Hildanus, the father of German surgery, or, as he has been sometimes called, the Ambroise Pare, of Germany, was also a contemporary of Harvey's. His real name was Fabry and he was born in Hilden, but he latinized his name into that form usually adopted today. Scultetus was another famous surgeon of the same period. William Gilbert, (1540-1603), had been the talented physician of Queen Elizabeth, and was among the first to study the experimental method. With the appearance of his book upon the magnet, in 1600, began the science of electricity and magnetism. He was the first to teach the fact that the earth itself was a great magnet and he distinguished between magnetic and electric reactions. Later the great Dutch anatomist, Ruysch, afforded corroboration of Harvey's views by another method, when he invented and practiced those beautiful minute injections of the vascular system which made him so famous, and built up that great collection of specimens which Peter the Great bought for Russia at an expense of about $75,000.

Contemporary with Harvey also was Swammerdam, one of the most versatile men of his time, famous as naturalist, savant, physiologist, linguist and poet. It was during the fifteenth century that astronomy began to assume an importance and degree of accuracy never hitherto known. This was due very largely to the independence of thought and the researches of Copernicus, who was born in Cremona in 1477, and who studied medicine in Krakau and astronomy in Vienna. He lived to the age of 70 and was the real father of the heliocentric theory, now known as the Copernican system, which he substituted for the previous Ptolemaic theory, thus reversing the ancient idea that the sun circled about the earth. Copernicus demonstrated the phases of the moon, but his opponents claimed that if this doctrine were true Venus would exhibit the same phenomena; to which he replied that it was true, though he knew not what to say to these objections, but that God was good and would in time furnish answer to them. It was Galileo's crude telescope which, in Harvey's younger day, in 1611, furnished this answer and revealed the phases of Venus. To illustrate how the views of Copernicus were received we might add here that Martin Luther paid his compliments to him by declaring that Copernicus was a fool who wished to stand astronomy upon its head.

Copernicus was succeeded by Galileo, who was born in 1554 in Pisa, and died 1642. He may be called the creator of dynamic astronomy and mechanics, as well as one of the most brilliant exponents of experimental and inductive reasoning. He was of noble birth and was, in fact, the torch bearer of physics at the period of The Renaissance. He gave up speculation and substituted for it the habit of observation, reaping a large harvest of surprising facts, any one of which might have immortalized him. He not only established the movements of the earth on its own axis as well as around the sun, which Copernicus had shown, but he discovered the weight of the atmosphere and first calculated the law of gravity. He and his successors were governed always by that aphorism which is today as true as ever: "Experience is deceptive and judgment difficult."

In 1615 when he was before The Inquisition, at Rome, and when its theologians had examined statements extracted from his letters, they solemnly rendered their decision in these words: "The first proposition that the sun is the center and does not revolve about the earth is foolish, absurd, false in theology and heretical, because expressly contrary to The Holy Scripture.

THE EVIL EYE

The second proposition that the earth is not the center, but revolves about the sun, is absurd, false in philosophy and, from a theological point of view, at least, opposed to the true faith."

This for a *pronunciamento* from the infallible Church! Galileo and Bruno have by some writers both been made to stand in an unpleasant light because of their recantation or shifting position before The Inquisition. Bruno was the greatest philosopher and skeptic of the latter part of the 16th century, and had outlined, withal somewhat vaguely, that which is now known as the nebular hypothesis. He was murdered by The Inquisition in 1600, and the views which he enunciated seem to have been buried with him, not to reappear until long after his sad fate had been consummated. He had, for instance, contended for the truths of the Copernican doctrine, but it was not until ten years after his martyrdom that Galileo proved it with his telescope. That both these great men yielded in some respects to the influences of The Inquisition and renounced some of their scientific "heresies" is largely to be excused by the fact that they were both old, broken in health from the sufferings which they had endured, as well as from their disappointments, and that they had been, under these circumstances, handed over to that Inquisition which knew no mercy. Galileo could well remember the *auto da fe* In the Piazza del Fiore, in Rome, the scene of Bruno's martyrdom, as well as the tragic end of many another who had dared to have the courage of his convictions. Let us, then, not judge him harshly, but be grateful even that the enormous power of The Inquisition did not and could not suppress the truth.

Galileo's discovery of the satellites of Jupiter, the rings of Saturn, his experiments with the pendulum, his construction of the telescope, as well as of the thermometer, and many other deeds, have stamped him as one of the great figures in the history of progress and science. It Is most interesting to note that this contemporary of Harvey's, like himself, was given to Inductions obtained from experimental studies. Another great astronomical light of Harvey's time was Keppler, who was driven from one place to another by religious fanaticism, until he ended his life in 1630. It was he who formulated the great principle which underlies the motions of the planets, and who gave to the world his so-called "laws," which so materially advanced the science of astronomy. It was he who really discovered that comet which was later given Halley's name, whose periodic return he first foretold. Such was the spirit of the times in which Harvey lived, and such the influences which surrounded his teachers before him and himself in turn. It makes a long preface to a consideration of what Harvey himself accomplished, but it is not without its interest because men and their deeds must be judged largely by their environment. Now, to speak more particularly of Harvey himself, and what was known of the circulation when he undertook his investigations.

The liver had been considered, from time immemorial, as the principal factor in the production and movement of the blood. The ancients supposed that here the veins took their origin and that through them the blood flowed to all parts of the body, returning to its source by an undulating movement or series of alternate waves. The arteries had been supposed to contain only vital spirits, whose great reservoir was the heart, although Erasistratus had admitted that in certain cases blood might escape into the arterial channels. Later Galen showed that the arteries always contained blood, and he knew that blood was poured into the right side of the heart by the great veins, but believed that only a little of it passed from the right ventricle into the lungs, the greater part of it passing through hypothetical pores in the septum and thus into the left ventricle. This opinion, like Galen's in other respects, remained unchanged until the middle of the 16th century. It was also known that valves existed within the veins, and that if an artery were tied on a living animal blood would cease to flow and pulsation be checked below the ligature, while if a vein were tied it shrunk above the ligature and became distended below.

THE EVIL EYE

Three men before Harvey's time came very near to discovering the secret that made him famous; in fact, they made such advances on what was already known that history should accord them a distinguished place. One was Columbus, who was born at Cremona in 1490, and died in 1559. He was first a pupil and prosector and then a friend of Vesalius, the great anatomist. Later he succeeded him at The University of Padua and unfortunately, after gaining his position, ungratefully turned upon his old teacher. He was, however, for his day a good anatomist and especially a good osteologist. It was he who first demonstrated experimentally that blood passes through the lungs into the pulmonary veins and that the latter connect with the left ventricle. He thus practically established the fact of the lesser circulation.

He suffered, however, as did Servetus, from the prevailing notion that spirits and blood were mixed together. From Padua Columbus went to Pisa, and then to Rome. He wrote with elegance and correctness of style and even described the vessels which penetrate the bone cells, the ossicles of the ear, the minute anatomy of the teeth, the ventricles of the larynx, as well as those valves which prevent the return of blood from the lungs to the heart. In fact, he narrowly missed the significance of the actual facts of the case, simply failing in his final analysis and assembling of those facts which he had already demonstrated.

Cesalpinus, who lived a little later, came still nearer the mark, having accepted the teachings of Columbus regarding the course of the blood through the lungs. He added that the ultimate arterial branches connect with those of the veins, and he taught that blood and vital spirits, from which the ancients could never separate themselves, passed from the arteries into the veins during sleep, as was demonstrated by the swelling of the veins and the diminution of the pulse at that time. A little later came Michael Servetus, who figures principally in history as a theologian and a victim of theologians, since he perished a martyr to Calvin's jealousy. He was, in effect, a wisely and widely educated man who did a great deal for science, one of the offenses attributed to him being an edition of Ptolemy's geography, in which Judea was described as a barren and inhospitable land instead of one "flowing with milk and honey."

This simple statement of a geographical fact was made a tremendous weapon of offense by Calvin, who replied that even if Servetus had only quoted from Ptolemy and, although there were ample geographical proofs, it nevertheless "unnecessarily inculpated Moses and grievously outraged The Holy Ghost." Servetus dared to deny the passage of the blood through the septum of the heart, and contended that that which comes into the right side was distributed to the lung and returned to the left ventricle. He published his views, however, in a religious treatise on errors concerning The Trinity, a most unfortunate place in which to inject such an important fact, since it gave his enemies a still greater opportunity to vent and ventilate their spleen. Had he been able to leave out that notion of vital spirits, which prevailed with all his predecessors, he might actually have made the great discovery left for Harvey to enunciate. I have not been able to refer to original documents In this matter, but it is claimed by some that his description of the circulation was contained In another religious work concerning the Restitution of Christianity, which was printed in Nuremburg In 1790.

Such was the actual state of knowledge concerning the movements of the blood and the functions of the heart when Harvey published his great work. It behooves us now to proceed with a short account of Harvey's own life and researches.

William Harvey was born at Folkstone on the first of April, 1578. He was the eldest son of a prosperous merchant who raised a large family and who occupied the highest positions of honor in his own town. The son William was born to his second wife, by whom he had seven sons and two daughters. All of these children were helped to remunerative or honorable positions. They became merchants or politicians or secured prominence in some way, but William was the only one to study medicine. He was sent to the King's school at Canterbury, In 1588, and he was admitted at Caius, in Cambridge, In 1593, where he graduated In arts in 1597. The following year he went to Padua, which then had one of the greatest medical schools of the time, and he obtained his medical diploma in 1602, when twenty-four years of age. Returning to England he received a doctor's degree at Cambridge, and shortly afterward married a daughter of a London physician and entered upon the practice of medicine in London. In the great city his practice as a physician seems to have been from the outset successful, and his knowledge and ability procured him various valuable appointments.

He was made a Fellow of The College of Physicians in 1607. This Royal College of Physicians was given a grant of incorporation by Henry VIII in 1518, at the intercession of Chambers, Linacre and Ferdinand Victoria, the King's Physicians, it being under the patronage of Cardinal Woolsey. The first meetings were held at Linacre's house which he bequeathed to the corporation at his death. Until this College was founded practitioners of medicine were licensed to practice by the Bishop of London or by the Dean of St. Paul's. A few years later Harvey was appointed Physician-extraordinary to King James I, and later yet, after the publication of his great treatise and its dedication to the King, he was made Physician-in-ordinary to Charles I, whom he attended during the Civil Wars.

It must have been about 1615 when Harvey first began expounding his views on the circulation of the blood, during lectures which were delivered at The College of Physicians, but it was not until thirteen years later, i, e, in 1628, that his great work DE MOTU CORDIS was published in Latin, as was customary among scholars, and at Frankfort-on-the-Main, since that was then the great center of the book publishing trade.

The treatise was dedicated to King Charles I, in a manner which to us would seem servile, and yet which was according to a custom followed by nearly all of the scholars of the day, who desired to attract not only the attention of royalty, but, in most instances, their benevolent assistance. It is worth while to quote at this point the first sentence or two of his dedication:

"To the
Most Serene and Invincible
CHARLES,
of Great Britain, France and Ireland,
KING: DEFENDER of the FAITH,
Most Serene King:

"The heart of animals is the basis of their life, the principle of the whole, the Sun of their Microcosm, that upon which all movement depends, from which all strength proceeds. The King in like manner is the basis of his Kingdom, the Sun of his World, the heart of the Commonwealth, whence all power derives, all grace appears. What I have here written of the movements of the heart I am the more emboldened to present to your Majesty, according to the Custom of the present age, because nearly all things human are done after human examples and many things In the King are after the pattern of the heart."

The dedication was followed by a Proemium which one may hardly read today without emotion. In it he sets forth the mystery that has surrounded the subject of the motion and function of the heart, as well as the attendant difficulties of the subject, speaking of his own early despair that he would ever be able to clear up the subject. He even said that at one time he found the matter so beset with difficulties that he was inclined to agree with Fracastorius "that the movements of the heart and their purpose could be comprehended by God alone." Only later was this despair dispelled by a suggestion when, as he says: "I began to think whether there might not be a movement in a circle" when thus the truth dawned fully upon him.

THE EVIL EYE

We shall have to speak later of the opposition provoked by the appearance of this work and its almost general rejection. It is perhaps, however, but just to those who disputed Harvey's discoveries to recall that no complete and actual demonstration of the actual circulation was possible at that time, nor for many years after, and until the introduction of the microscope, the common magnifying glass of that day being the only lens in use. It remained for Malpighi to demonstrate the blood actually in circulation In the lung of a frog some three or four years after Harvey's death. In 1657. But Harvey lived long enough to see his views gain general acceptance, and though at first, and as the result of the opposition provoked by his publication, his practice fell off mightily, he later regained his professional position and rose to the highest eminence, being elected In 1654 to the Presidency of the College of Physicians. To this institution he proved a great benefactor, making considerable additions to the building after its destruction in The Great Fire of 1666 and its subsequent restoration.

He also left a certain sum of money as a foundation for an annual oration, to be delivered in commemoration of those who had been great benefactors of the College. This oration is still regularly delivered on St. Luke's Day, i. e., the 18th of October, and is ordinarily known as the Harveian oration. In these orations more or less reference to Harvey's work and influence is always made. This great man passed away on the 3rd of June, 1657, within ten months of his eightieth birthday, thus affording a brilliant exception to the list of men who have rendered great service to the world and not lived long enough to see it appreciated. As one reads Harvey's own words, the wonder ever grows that it should have remained for him, after the lapse of so many centuries, to not only call attention to what had been said by Galen but apparently forgotten by his successors, namely, that "the arteries contained blood and nothing but blood, and, consequently, neither spirits nor air, as may be readily gathered from experiments and reasonings," which he elsewhere furnishes. He furthermore shows how Galen demonstrated this by applying two ligatures upon an exposed artery at some distance from each other, and then opening the vessel itself in which nothing but blood could be found. He calls attention also to the result of ligation of one of the large vessels of an extremity, the inevitable result being just what we today know it must be, and the procedure terminating with gangrene of the limb.

Not long before Harvey's own publication, Fabricius, he of Aquapendente, had published a work on respiration, stating that, as the pulsation of the heart and arteries was insufficient for the ventilation and refrigeration of the blood, therefore were the lungs fashioned to surround the heart. Harvey showed how the arterial pulse and respiration could not serve the same ends, combating the view generally held, that if the arteries were filled with air, a larger quantity of air penetrating when the pulse is large and full, it must come to pass that if one plunge into a bath of water or of oil when the pulse is strong and full it should forthwith become either smaller or much slower, since the surrounding fluid would render it either difficult or impossible for air to penetrate. He also called attention to the inconsistencies between this view and the arrangement of the prenatal circulation; also to the fact that marine animals, living in the depths of the sea, could under no circumstances take in or emit air by the movements of their arteries and beneath the infinite mass of waters, inasmuch as "to say that they absorb the air that is present in the water and emit their fumes into this medium, were to utter something very like a figment;" furthermore "when the windpipe is divided, air enters and returns through the wound by two opposite movements, but when an artery is divided blood escapes in one continuous stream and no air passes."

Discussing further the views which he stigmatized as so incongruous and mutually subversive that every one of them is justly brought under suspicion, he reverts again to the statements of Galen, calling attention to the fact that from a single divided artery the whole of the blood of the body may be withdrawn in the course of half an hour or less, and to the inevitable consequences of such an act; also that when an artery is opened the blood is emptied with force and in jets, and that the impulse corresponds with that of the heart; again that In an aneurysm the pulsation is the same as in other arteries, appealing for corroboration in this matter to the recent statements of Riolan, who later became his avowed enemy. Harvey also called attention to the fact that while ordinarily there was a seemingly fixed relation between respiration and pulserate, this might vary very much under certain circumstances, showing that respiration and circulation were two totally different processes. Harvey utilized also the results of his researches in comparative anatomy and physiology, for early in his work he called attention to the fact that every animal which is unfurnished with lungs lacks a right ventricle.

In his Proemlum he then proceeds to ask certain very pertinent questions which can only be briefly summarized in this place. He asks: First, why, inasmuch as the structure of both ventricles is practically identical, it should be imagined that their uses are different, and why, if tricuspid valves are placed at the entrance into the right ventricle and prove obstacles to the return of blood into vena cava, and if similar valves are situated at the commencement of the pulmonary artery, preventing return of blood into the ventricle, then why, when similar valves are found in connection with the other side of the heart, should we deny that they are there for the same purpose of prevention "here the egress" and "there the regurgitation of the blood?"

Secondly, he asks why, in view of the similarity of these structures, it should be said that things are arranged in the left ventricle for the egress and regress of spirits, and in the right ventricle for those of blood?

Thirdly, he inquires why, when one notes the resemblance between the passages and vessels connected with the opposite sides of the heart, one should regard one side as destined to a private purpose, namely, that of nourishing the lungs, the other to a more public function? Furthermore, he inquires, since the lungs are so near, and in continual movement, and the vessels supplying them of such dimensions, what can be the use of the pulse of the right ventricle, which he had often observed in the course of his experiments?

He sums up his inability to accept the explanations previously offered with a phrase which reads rather strangely, even in original Latin: "Deus bone! Quomodo tricuspides impediunt aeris egressum, non sanguinis." i. e., "'Good God! how should the mitral valves prevent the regurgitation of air and not of blood?"

He then takes up the views of those who have believed that the blood oozed through the septum of the heart from the right to the left side by certain secret pores, and to them he replied "By Hercules, no such pores can be demonstrated, nor, in fact, do any such exist." Again, "Besides, if the blood could permeate the substance of the septum, or could be emptied from the ventricles, what use were there for the coronary artery and vein, branches of which proceed to the septum itself, to supply it with nourishment?"

Further on in the treatise Harvey sets forth his motives for writing, stating how greatly unsettled had become his mind in that he did not know what he himself should conclude nor what to believe from others. He says: "I was not surprised that Laurentius should have written that the movements of the heart were as perplexing as the flux and reflux of Euripus had appeared to Aristotle." He apologizes for the crime, as some of his friends considered it, that he should dare to depart from the precepts and opinions of all anatomists. He acknowledged that he took the step all the more willingly, seeing that Fabricius, who had accurately and learnedly delineated almost every one of the several parts of animals in a special work, had left the heart entirely untouched.

Passing more directly to the actual work of the heart, he shows that not only are the ventricles contracted by virtue of the muscular structure of their own walls, but further that those fibers or bands, styled "Nerves" by Aristotle, that are so conspicuous in the ventricles of larger animals when they contract simultaneously, by an admirable adjustment, help to draw together all the internal surfaces as if with cords, thus expelling the charge of contained blood with force. Later on he says that if the pulmonary artery be opened, blood will be seen spurting forth from it, just as when any other artery is punctured, and that the same result follows division of the vessel which in fishes leads from the heart. He furnishes a very happy simile to prove that the pulses of the arteries are due to the impulses of the left ventricle by showing how, when one blows into a glove all of its fingers will be found to have become distended at one and the same time. He quotes Aristotle, who made no distinction between veins and arteries, but said that the blood of all animals palpitates within their vessels and by the pulse is sent everywhere simultaneously, all of this depending upon the heart.

It is in Chapter Five of the treatise that he gives, probably for the first time, an accurate published account of just what transpires with one complete cycle of cardiac activity. The passage need not be quoted here, but deserves to be read by everyone interested in the subject, as who should not be? One sentence, however, is worth quotation or, at least, a summary, as follows: "But if the divine Galen will here allow, as in other places he does, that all the arteries of the body arise from the great artery, and that this takes its origin from the heart; that all the vessels naturally contain and carry blood; that the three semi-lunar valves situated at the orifice of the aorta prevent the return of the blood into the heart, and that they were here for some important purpose- I do not see how he can deny that the great artery is the very vessel to carry the blood, when it has attained its highest triumph of perfection, from the heart for distribution to all parts of the body."

His Chapter Six deals with the course by which blood is carried from the right into the left ventricle, and here one must admire the large number of experimental demonstrations which Harvey had undertaken upon all classes of animals, for he speaks even of that which occurs in small insects, whose circulation he had studied so far as he could with the simple lens. Furthermore he described the prenatal circulation, omitting practically nothing of that which is taught today, showing that in embryos, while the lungs are yet in a state of inaction, both ventricles of the heart are employed, as if they were but one, for the transmission of blood. In concluding this chapter he again states briefly the course of the blood, and promises to show, first, that this may be so and, then, to prove that it really is so.

His Chapter Seven is devoted to showing how the blood passes through the substance of the lungs from the right ventricle and then on into the pulmonary vein and left ventricle. He alludes to the multitude of doubters as belonging, as the poet had said, to that race of men who, when they will, assent full readily, and when they will not, by no matter of means; who, when their assent is wanted, fear, and when it is not, fear not to give it. A little later on he says: "As there are some who admit nothing unless upon authority, let them learn that the truth I am contending for can be confirmed from Galen's own words, namely, that not only may the blood be transmitted from the pulmonary artery into the pulmonary veins and then into the left ventricle of the heart, but that this is effected by the ceaseless pulsation of the heart and the movements of the lungs in breathing." He then shows how Galen explained the uses of the valves and the necessity for their existence, as well as the universal mutual anastomosis of the arteries with the veins, and that the heart is incessantly receiving and expelling blood by and from its ventricles, for which purpose it is furnished with four sets of valves, two for escape and two for inlet and their regulation.

Harvey then noted a well-known clinical fact, that the

more frequent or forcible the pulsations, the more speedily might the body be deprived of its blood during hemorrhage, and that it thus happens that in fainting fits and the like, when the heart beats more languidly, hemorrhages are diminished and arrested. The balance of the book is practically devoted to further demonstration and corroboration of statements already made. A study of this work of Harvey's illustrates how much respect even he and his contemporaries still showed for the authority of Galen. It shows still further how nearly Galen came to the actual truth concerning the circulation. Had the latter not adopted too many of the notions of his predecessors concerning the nature of the soul (Anima) and the spirits (Pneuma) of man, he might himself have anticipated Harvey by a thousand years, and by such announcement of a great truth have set forward physiology by an equal period. Independent and original as Harvey showed himself, he seems to have failed to get away from the notion of the vapors and spiritual nature of the blood which he had inherited from the writings of Galen and many others. Nevertheless he also alludes to this same blood as alimentive and nutritive. We must not forget, however, that this was years before Priestly's discovery of oxygen and that Harvey had, like others, no notion of the actual purpose of the lungs, believing that the purification and revivification of the blood was the office of the heart itself.

Along with its other intrinsic merits Harvey's book possesses a clear and logical arrangement, the author first disposing of the errors of antiquity, describing next the behavior of the heart in the living animal, showing its automatic pumplike structure, its alternate contractions and the other phenomena already alluded to, thus piling up facts one upon another In a manner which proved quite irresistible. The only thing that he missed was the ultimate connection between the veins and the arteries, i. e., the capillaries, which it remained for Malpighi to discover with the then new and novel microscope, which he did about 1657, showing the movement of the blood cells in the small vessels, and confirming the reality of that ultimate communication which had been held to exist. Malpighi discovered the blood corpuscles in 1665, but it remained for Leeuwenhoek, of Delft, in 1690, by using an improved instrument to demonstrate to all observers the actual movements of the circulating blood in the living animal. One historian has said that with Harvey's overthrow of the old teachings regarding the importance of the liver and of the spirits in the heart "fell the four fundamental humors and qualities" while Daremberg exclaims: "As in one of the days of the creation, chaos disappeared and light was separated from darkness."

It remains now only to briefly consider how Harvey's great discovery was received. To quote the words of one writer: "So much care and circumspection in search for truth, so much modesty and firmness In its demonstration, so much clearness and method in the development of his Ideas, should have prepossessed everyone in favor of the theory of Harvey; on the contrary, it caused a general stupefaction in the medical world and gave rise to great opposition." During the quarter of a century which elapsed after Harvey's announcement there probably was not an anatomist nor physiologist of any prominence who did not take active part in the controversy engendered by it; even the philosopher Descartes was one of the first adherents of the doctrine of the circulation, which he corroborated by experiments of his own.

Two years after the appearance of Harvey's book appeared an attack, composed in fourteen days by one Primerose, a man of Scotch descent, born and educated in France, but practicing at Hull, in which he pronounced the impossibilities of surpassing the ancients or improving on the work of Riolan, who already had written in opposition to Harvey, and who was the only one to whom the latter vouchsafed an answer. It was Riolan who procured a decree of the Faculty of Paris prohibiting the teaching of Harvey's doctrine. It was this same Riolan who combated with equal violence and obstinacy the other great discovery of the age, namely, the circulation of the lymph.

One of the earliest and fiercest adversaries of Harvey's theory was Plempius, of Louvaine, who, however, gave way to the force of argument and who finally publicly and voluntarily passed over to the ranks of its defenders in 1652, becoming one of Harvey's most enthusiastic advocates. Harvey's conduct through the controversy was always of the most dignified character; in fact, he rarely ventured to reply in any way to his adversaries, believing in the ultimate triumph of the truths which he had enunciated. His only noteworthy reply was one addressed to Riolan, then Professor in the Paris Faculty and one of the greatest anatomists of his age, to whose opinion great value was always attached. Even in debating or arguing against him, Harvey always spoke of him with great deference, calling him repeatedly The Prince of Science. Riolan was, however, never converted, though whether he held to his previous position from obstinacy, from excess of respect for the ancients, or from envy and jealousy of his contemporary, is not known. Another peculiar spectacle was afforded by one Parisunus, who died in 1643, physician in Venice, who, like Harvey, had been a pupil of Fabricius of Aquapendente, who had been stigmatized by Riolan as an ignoramus in anatomy, but who joined with others in declaring that he had seen the heart beat when perfectly bloodless, and that no beating of the heart and no sounds were to be heard as Harvey had affirmed. With the later and more minute studies into the structure and function of the heart we are not here concerned. The endeavor has been rather to place before you the sentiments, the knowledge and the habits of thought of the men of Harvey's time, with the briefest possible epitome of what they knew, or rather of how little they knew, to account for this later slavish adherence to authority by unwillingness to reason independently, or to observe natural phenomena intelligently, still less to experiment with them. It is, then, rather the brief history of an epochal discovery than an effort to trace out its far-reaching consequences that I have endeavored to give.

THE EVIL EYE

Here must close an account which perhaps has been to you tedious, and yet which is really brief, of Harvey's life and labors. He lived to see his views generally accepted and to enjoy his own triumph, a pleasure not attained by many great inventors or discoverers. Lessons of great importance may be gathered from a more careful study of this great historical epoch, but they must be left to your own powers of reasoning rather than to what I may add here. I commend it to you as a fertile source of inspiration, and a line of research worthy of both admiration and imitation. Few men have rendered greater service to the world by the shedding of blood than did Harvey, in his innocent and wonderful studies of its natural movement. Perhaps it might be said of him that he was the first man to show that "blood will tell." What he made it tell has been thus briefly told to you.

I know not how I may better close this account than by quoting the concluding words of his famous book, and especially repeating the lines which he has quoted from some Latin author whom I have not been able to identify. His paragraph and his quotation are as follows:

"Finally, if any use or benefit to this department of the republic of letters should accrue from my labors, it will, perhaps, be allowed that I have not lived idly, and, as the old man in the comedy says:

'For never yet hath anyone attained
To such perfection, but that time, and place.
And use, have brought addition to his knowledge;
Or made correction, or admonished him.
That he was ignorant of much which he
Had thought he knew; or led him to reject
What he had once esteemed of highest price.'"

XIII: HISTORY OF ANAESTHESIA AND THE INTRODUCTION OF ANAESTHETICS IN SURGERY

IN COMMEMORATION OF THE SEMI-CENTENNIAL OF THE INTRODUCTION OF ETHER AS AN ANAESTHETIC AGENT

Commemorative Address delivered at the Medical Department, University of Buffalo, October 16, 1896.

Fifty years ago today- that is to say, on the 16th of October, 1846- there occurred an event which marks as distinct a step in human progress as almost any that could be named by the erudite historian. I refer to the first demonstration of the possibility of alleviating pain during surgical operations. Had this been the date of a terrible battle, on land or sea, with mutual destruction of thousands of human beings, the date itself would have been signalized in literature and would have been impressed upon the memory of every schoolboy, while the names of the great military murderers who commanded the opposing armies would have been emblazoned upon monuments and the pages of history. But this event was merely the conquest of pain and the alleviation of human suffering, and no one who has ever served his race by contributing to either of these results has been remembered beyond his own generation or outside the circle of his immediate influence. Such is the irony of fate. The world erects imposing monuments or builds tombs, like that of Napoleon, to the memory of those who have been the greatest destroyers of their race; and so Caesar, Hannibal, Genghis Khan, Richard the Lion-hearted, Gustavus Vasa, Napoleon and hundreds of other great military murderers have received vastly more attention, because of their race-destroying propensities and abilities, than if they had ever fulfilled fate in any other capacity. But the men like Sir Spencer Wells, who has added his 40,000 years of life to the total of human longevity, or like Sir Joseph Lister, who has shown our profession how to conquer that arch enemy of time past, surgical sepsis, or like Morton, who first publicly demonstrated how to bring on a safe and temporary condition of insensibility to pain, are men more worthy in our eyes of lasting fame, and much greater heroes of their times, and of all time- yet are practically unknown to the world at large, to whom they have ministered in such an unmistakable and superior way.

This much, then, by way of preface and reason for commemorating in this public way the semi-centennial of this really great event. Because the world does scant honor to these men we should be all the more mindful of their services, and all the more insistent upon their public recognition. Of all the achievements of the Anglo-Saxon race, I hold it true that the two greatest and most beneficent were the discovery of ether and the introduction of antiseptic methods- one of which we owe to an American, the other to a Briton. The production of deep sleep and the usual accompanying abolition of pain have been subjects which have ever appeared, in some form, in myth or fable, and to which poets of all times have alluded, usually with poetic license. One of the most popular of these fables connects the famous oracle of Apollo, at Delphi, whence proceeded mysterious utterances and inchoate sounds, with convulsions, delirium and insensibility upon the part of those who approached it. To what extent there is a basis of fact in this tradition can never be explained, but it is not improbable from what we now know of hypnotic influence.

From all time it has been known that many different plants and herbs contained principles which were narcotic, stupefying or intoxicating. These properties have especially been ascribed to the juices of the poppy, the deadly nightshade, henbane, the Indian hemp and the mandragora, which for us now is the true mandrake, whose juice has long been known as possessing soporific influence. Ulysses and his companions succumbed to the influence of Nepenthe; and, nineteen hundred years ago, when crucifixion was a common punishment of malefactors, it was customary to assuage their last hours upon the cross by a draught of vinegar with gall or myrrh, which had real or supposititious narcotic properties. Even the prophet Amos, seven hundred years before the time of Christ, spoke of such a mixture as this as "the wine of the condemned," for he says, in rehearsing the iniquities of Israel by which they had incurred the anger of the Almighty: "And they lay themselves down upon the clothes laid to pledge by every altar, and they drink the wine of the condemned in the house of their God," (Chap. II, verse 8), meaning thereby undoubtedly that these people, in their completely demoralized condition, drank the soporific draught kept for criminals. Herodotus mentions a habit of the Scythians, who employed a vapor generated from the seed of the hemp for the purpose of producing an intoxication by inhalation.

Narcotic lotions were also used for bathing the people about to be operated upon. Pliny, who perished at the destruction of Herculaneum, A. D. 79, testified to the soporific power of the preparations made from mandragora upon the faculties of those who drank it. He says: "It is drunk against serpents and before cuttings and puncturings, lest they should be felt." He also describes the indifference to pain produced by drinking a vinous infusion of the seeds of eruca, called by us the rocket, upon criminals about to undergo punishment. Dioscorides relates of mandragora that "some boil down the roots in wine to a third part, and preserve the juice thus procured, and give one cyathus of this to cause the insensibility of those who are about to be cut or cauterized." One of his later commentators also states that wine in which mandragora roots have been steeped "does bring on sleep and appease pain, so that it is given to those who are to be cut, sawed or burnt in any parts of their body, that they may not perceive pain."

Apuleius, about a century later than Pliny, advised the use of the same preparation. The Chinese, in the earlier part of the century, gave patients preparations of hemp, by which they became completely insensible and were operated upon in many ways. This hemp is the cannabis Indica which furnishes the Hasheesh of the Orient and the intoxicating and deliriating Bhang, about which travelers in the East used to write so much. In Barbara, for instance, it was always taken if possible, by criminals condemned to suffer mutilation or death.

According to the testimony of medieval writers, knowledge of these narcotic drugs was practically applied during the last of the Crusades, the probability being that the agent principally employed was this same hasheesh. Hugo di Lucca gave a complete formula for the preparation of the mixture, with which a sponge was to be saturated, dried, and then, when wanted, was to be soaked in warm water, and afterward applied to the nostrils, until he who was to be operated upon had fallen asleep; after which he was aroused with the vapor of vinegar. Strangely enough, the numerous means of attaining insensibility, then more or less known to the common people, and especially to criminals and executioners, do not appear to have found favor for use during operations. Whether this was due to unpleasant aftereffects, or from what reason, we are not informed.

Only one or two surgical writers beside Guy de Chaullac (1498) refer In their works to agents for relief of pain, and then almost always to their unpleasant effects, the danger of producing asphyxiation, and the like. Ambrose Pare wrote that preparations of mandragora were formerly used to avert pain. In 1579, an English surgeon, Bulleyn, affirmed that it was possible to put the patient into an anesthetic state during the operation of lithotomy, but spoke of It as a "terrible dream." One Meisner spoke of a secret remedy used by Weiss, about the end of the XVII Century, upon Augustus II., king of Poland, who produced therewith such perfect insensibility to pain that an amputation of the royal foot was made without suffering, even without royal consent. The advice which the Friar gave Juliet regarding the distilled liquor which she was to drink, and which should presently throw her Into a cold and drowsy humor, although a poetic generality, is Shakespeare's recognition of a popular belief. Middleton, a tragic writer of Shakespeare's day, in his tragedy known as "Women beware Women," refers in the following terms to anesthesia In surgery:

> "I'll imitate the pities of old surgeons
> To this lost limb, who, ere they show their art.
> Cast one asleep; then cut the diseased part."

Of course, of all the narcotics in use by educated men, opium has been, since its discovery and introduction, the most popular and generally used. Surgeons of the last century were accustomed to administer large doses of it shortly before an operation, which, if serious, was rarely performed until the opiate effect was manifested. Still, in view of its many unpleasant after-effects, its use was restricted, so far as possible, to extreme cases. Baron Larrey, noticing the benumbing effect of cold upon wounded soldiers, suggested its introduction for anesthetic purposes, and Arnott, of London, systematized the practice, by recommending a freezing mixture of ice and salt to be laid directly upon the part to be cut. Other surgeons were accustomed to put their patients into a condition of either alcoholic intoxication or alcoholic stupor. Long-continued compression of a part was also practiced by some, by which a limb could, as we say, be made to "go to sleep." A few others recommended to produce faintness by excessive bleeding. It was in 1776 that the arch-fraud Mesmer entered Paris and began to initiate people into the mysteries of what he called animal magnetism, which was soon named mesmerism, after him.

Thoroughly degenerate and disreputable as he was, he nevertheless taught people some new truths, which many of them learned to their sorrow, while in the hospitals of France and England severe operations were performed upon patients thrown into a mesmeric trance, and without suffering upon their part. That a scientific study of the mesmeric phenomena has occupied the attention of eminent men in recent years, and that hypnotism is now recognized as an agent often capable of producing insensibility to pain is simply true, as these facts have been turned to the real benefit of man by scientific students rather than by quacks and charlatans. In 1799, Sir Humphrey Davey, being at that time an assistant in the private hospital of Dr. Beddoes, which was established for treatment of disease by inhalation of gases, and which he called The Pneumatic Institute, began experimenting with nitrous oxide gas, and noticed Its exhilarating and intoxicating effects; also the relief from pain which it afforded in headache and toothache. As the results of his reports, a knowledge of Its properties was diffused all over the world, and it was utilized both for amusement and exhibition purposes. Davey even wrote as follows of this gas:

"As nitrous oxide. In its extensive operation, appears capable of destroying physical pain, it may probably be used with advantage during surgical operations in which no great effusion of blood takes place." It is not at all unlikely that Colton and Wells, to be soon referred to, derived encouragement, if not incentive, from these statements of Davey. Nevertheless, Velpeau, perhaps the greatest French surgeon of his day, wrote in 1839, that "to escape pain In surgical operations is a chimera which we are not permitted to look for in our day."

Sulfuric ether, as a chemical compound, was known from the XIII Century, for reference was made to it by Raymond LuUy. It was first spoken of by the name of ether by Godfrey, in the Transactions of the London Royal Society, In 1730, while Isaac Newton spoke of it as the ethereal spirits of wine. During all of the previous century it was known as a drug, and allusion to its inhalation was made in 1795 in a pamphlet, probably by Pearson. Beddoes, In 1796, stated that "It gives almost immediate relief, both to the oppression and pain in the chest. In cases of pectoral catarrh." In 1815, Nysten spoke of inhalation of ether as being common treatment for mitigating pain in colic, and in 1816 he described an Inhaler for its use. As early as 1812 it was often inhaled for experiment or amusement, and so-called "ether frolics" were common in various parts of the country.

This was true, particularly for our purpose, of the students of Cambridge, and of the common people in Georgia in the vicinity of Long's home. It probably is for this reason that a host of claimants for the honor of the discovery appeared so soon as the true anesthetic properties of the drug were demonstrated. There probably is every reason to think that, either by accident or design, a condition of greater or less insensibility to pain had been produced between 1820 and 1846, by a number of different people, educated and ignorant, but that no one had the originality or the hardihood to push these investigations to the point of determining the real usefulness of ether. This was partly from ignorance, partly from fear, and partly because of the generally accepted impossibility of producing safe insensibility to pain. So, while independent claims sprang up from various sources, made by aspirants for honors in this direction, it is undoubtedly as properly due to Morton to credit him with the introduction of this agent as an anesthetic as to credit Columbus with the discovery of the New World, in spite of certain evidences that some portions of the American continent had been touched upon by adventurous voyagers before Columbus ever saw it.

The noun "anesthesia" and the adjective "anesthetic" were suggestions of Dr. Oliver Wendell Holmes, who early proposed their use to Dr. Morton in a letter which is still preserved. He suggests them with becoming modesty, advises Dr. Morton to consult others before adopting them, but, nevertheless, states that he thinks them apt for that purpose. The word anesthesia, therefore, is just about of the same age as the condition itself, and it, too, deserves commemoration upon this occasion. As one reads the history of anesthesia, which has been written up by a number of different authors, each, for the main part, having some particular object in view, or some particular friend whose claims he wishes especially to advocate, he may find mentioned at least a dozen different names of men who are supposed to have had more or less to do with this eventful discovery. But, for all practical purposes, one may reduce the list of claimants for the honor to four men, each of whose claims I propose to briefly discuss. These men were Long, Wells, Jackson and Morton. Of these four, two were dentists and two practicing physicians, to whom fate seems to have been unkind, as it often is, since three of them at least died a violent or distressing death, while the fourth lived to a ripe old age, harassed at almost every turn by those who sought to decry his reputation or injure his fortunes.

Crawford W. Long was born in Danielsville, Ga., in 1816. In 1839 he graduated from the Medical Department of the University of Pennsylvania. In the part of the country where Long settled it was a quite common occurrence to have what were known as "ether frolics" at social gatherings, ether being administered to various persons to the point of exhilaration, which in some instances was practically uncontrollable. Long's friends claim that he had often noticed that when the ether effect was pushed to this extent the subjects of the frolic became oblivious to minor injuries, and that these facts, often noticed, suggested to his mind the use of ether in surgical operations.

There is good evidence to show that Long first administered ether for this purpose on the 30th of March, 1842, and that on June 6th he repeated this performance upon the same patient; that In July he amputated a toe for a negro boy, but that the fourth operation was not performed until September of 1843. In 1844 a young man, named Wilhite, who had helped to put a colored boy to sleep at an ether frolic in 1839, became a student of Dr. Long's, to whom Long related his previous experiences. Long had never heard of Wilhite's episode, but had only one opportunity, in 1845, to try it, again upon a negro boy. Long lived at such a distance from railroad communication (130 miles) as to have few advantages, either of practice, observation or access to literature. Long made no public mention of his use of ether until 1849, when he published An Account of the First Use of Sulfuric Ether by Inhalation as an Anesthetic in Surgical

Operations, stating that he first read of Morton's experiments in an editorial in the Medical Examiner of December, 1846, and again later; on reading which articles he determined to wait before publishing any account of his own discovery, to see whether anyone else would present a prior claim. No special attention was paid to Long's article, as it seemed that he merely desired to place himself on record. There is little, probably no reasonable doubt as to Long's priority in the use of ether as an anesthetic, although it is very doubtful if he carried it, at least at first, to Its full extent. Nevertheless Long was an isolated observer, working entirely by himself, having certainly no opportunity and apparently little ambition to announce his discovery, and having no share in the events by which the value of ether was made known to the world. Long's strongest advocate was the late Dr. Marion Sims, who made a strong plea for his friend, and yet was not able to successfully establish anything more than has just been stated. As Dr. Morton's son, Dr. W. J. Morton, of New York, says, when writing of his father's claim: "Men used steam to propel boats before Fuller; electricity to convey messages before Morse; vaccine virus to avert smallpox before Jenner; and ether to annul pain before Morton."

But these men are not generally credited with their introduction by the world at large and, he argues, neither should Long or the other contestants be given the credit due Morton himself. In fact. Long writes of his own work that the result of his second experiment was such as to make him conclude that ether would only be applicable in cases where its effects could be kept up by constant use; in other words, that the anesthetic state was of such short duration that it was to him most unsatisfactory. Sir James Paget has summed up the relative claims of our four contestants in an article entitled Escape from Pain, published in the Nineteenth Century for December, 1879. He says:

"While Long waited, and Wells turned back, and Jackson was thinking, and those to whom they had talked were neither acting nor thinking, Morton, the practical man, went to work and worked resolutely. He gave ether successfully in severe surgical operations; he loudly proclaimed his deeds and he compelled mankind to hear him."

Horace Wells was born in Hartford, Vt., in 1815. In 1834 he began to study dentistry in Boston, and after completing his studies began to practice in Hartford, Ct. He was a man of no small ingenuity, and devised many novelties for his work. In December, 1844, he listened to a lecture delivered by Dr. Colton, who took for his subject nitrous oxide gas, the amusing effects of which he demonstrated to his audience upon a number of persons who visited the platform for that purpose. Wells was one of these. Wells, moreover, noticed that another young man, who bruised himself while under its influence, said afterward that he had not hurt himself at all. Wells then stated to a bystander that he thought that if one took enough of that kind of gas he could have a tooth extracted and not feel it. He at once called upon a neighboring dentist friend and made arrangements to test the anesthetic effects of the gas upon himself the next morning. Accordingly Colton gave him the gas, and Riggs, the friend, extracted the tooth; and Wells, returning to consciousness, assured them both that he had not suffered a particle of pain. He began at once to construct an apparatus for its manufacture. Dr. Marcey, of Hartford, then informed Wells that while a student at Amherst he and others had often inhaled nitrous oxide as well as the vapor of ether, for amusement, and suggested to Wells to try ether. After a few trials, however, it was found more difficult to administer, and Wells accordingly resolved to adhere to gas alone. This was in 1844, two years after Long's obscure experiments, of which, of course, they were ignorant. In 1845, Wells visited Boston for the purpose of introducing his discovery, and among others called upon his former partner, Morton, trying to establish the use of the gas. He soon became discouraged, however, and returned to Hartford, resuming his practice. There he continued to use gas for about two years, but failed to secure its introduction into general surgery, owing to prejudice and ignorance on the part of dentists and physicians alike. Wells's claims have been advocated by many of his fellow-citizens, and In Bushnell Park, In Hartford, stands a monument erected by the city and the state, dedicated to Horace Wells, "who discovered anesthesia, November, 1844."

C. T. Jackson was born In Plymouth, Mass., In 1805. He graduated In the Harvard Medical School in 1829, after which he went abroad, where he remained for several years, made the acquaintance of the most distinguished men, experimented in general science, electricity and magnetism and even devised a telegraphic apparatus, similar to that which Morse patented a year later. Returning, In 1835, he opened in Boston a laboratory for instruction in analytical chemistry, the first of its kind in the country. He also made quite a reputation as a geologist and mineralogist and received official appointments from Maine, Rhode Island, New Hampshire and other states. In 1845 he discovered and opened up copper and iron mines in the Lake Superior district. In 1846 and 1847 he was much aroused by Morton's experiments with sulfuric ether, and claimed even that he had suggested the use of ether to Morton, claiming also that he had himself been relieved of an acute distress by inhalation of ether vapor, and that it was from reflection on the phenomena presented in his own case that the possibility of its use for relief of pain during surgical operations suggested itself to him. This led to a triangular conflict for the priority of discovery between Wells, Jackson and Morton, each claiming the honor for himself. Well's health soon gave way. He went abroad and got recognition from the French Institute and the Paris Academy of Sciences, which did not, however, endorse his claim as discoverer nor accept nitrous oxide as an anesthetic.

Wells returned to find that Morton was on the tide of popular favor, the public having endorsed ether as the only reliable anesthetic. His mind became unbalanced, and in a fit of temporary aberration he ended his own life in a prison cell, in New York city in 1848. Wells being out of the way, Jackson became Morton's most violent opponent, and the two indulged in a most bitter fight and unseemly discussion. A few years later, Jackson, who, as remarked, had an extensive acquaintance abroad, visited Europe and presented his claim to the credit of the discovery of ether before various individuals and learned bodies, and so well did he work upon the French Institute as to be recognized as the discoverer of modern anesthesia. A select committee of the House of Representatives, to whom in 1854 Congress referred the matter, announced the following conclusions:

"First, that Dr. Horace Wells did not make any discovery of the anesthetic properties of the vapor of ether which he himself considered reliable and which he thought proper to give to the world. That his experiments were confined to nitrous oxide, but did not show it to be an efficient and reliable anesthetic agent... Second, that Dr. Charles T. Jackson does not appear at any time to have made any discovery in regard to ether which was not in print in Great Britain some years before... Fifth, that the whole agency of Dr. Jackson in the matter appears to consist entirely in his having made certain suggestions to aid Dr. Morton to make the discovery."

In 1873, Jackson's mind gave way, and after seven years of confinement In an asylum he died in 1880, at the age of 75, having been the recipient of many honors from foreign potentates and learned societies. William T. G. Morton was born In Charleston, Mass., in 1819. After a disastrous experience in business he was sent to Baltimore in 1840 and began the study of dentistry. In 1841 he entered the dental office of Horace Wells as student and assistant, becoming a partner in 1842. In 1843 the partnership was dissolved, Wells removing to Hartford, as before stated. Morton, ambitious for a medical degree, entered his name as a student In the office of Charles T. Jackson, in 1844, and the same year matriculated in the Harvard Medical School, though he never graduated. Having learned through Wells of the latter's successful use of nitrous oxide gas, but not knowing how to make it, he sought the advice of Dr. Jackson, who informed him that its preparation entailed considerable difficulty, and inquired for what purpose he wanted it. On Morton's replying that he wished to use it to make patients insensible to pain, Jackson suggested the use of sulfuric ether, as Marcey had suggested it to Wells two years previously, saying that it would produce the same effect and did not require any apparatus. Jackson also told Morton of the ether frolics common at Cambridge among the students. That same evening, September 30, 1846, Morton administered ether to a patient and extracted a tooth for him without pain. The next day he visited the office of a patent lawyer, for the purpose of securing a patent upon the new discovery. This lawyer ascertained that Jackson had been intimately connected with its suggestion, and came to the conclusion that a patent could not safely issue to either one independently of the other. But Jackson being a member of the State Medical Society, against whose ethical code it is to patent discoveries that pertain to the welfare of patients, and fearing the censure of his colleagues, agreed at once to assign his right over to Morton, receiving in return a 10 percent commission upon all that the latter made out of it. Morton, as a dentist, having no more compunction then than dentists have now upon the securement of a patent- in other words, being actuated by no fine ethical scruples- secured the patent, and then called upon Dr. J. Mason Warren, one of the surgeons in the Massachusetts General Hospital. Warren promised his cooperation and appointed the 16th of October, 1846, for the first public trial. Upon this occasion the clinic room was filled with visitors and students, when Morton placed the young man under the influence of his "letheon," as he called it then; after which Warren removed a tumor from his neck. The trial was most successful. Another took place on the following day, and on November 7th an amputation and an excision of the jaw were made, both patients being under the influence of letheon and oblivious to pain. At this time the nature of the anesthetic agent was kept a secret, the vapor of ether being disguised by aromatics, so as not to be recognized by anyone present.

THE EVIL EYE

True to the highest traditions of their craft, the staff of the Massachusetts General Hospital now met and declined to make further use of a drug whose composition was thus kept secret. It was then that Morton revealed the exact nature of it as sulfuric ether, disguised with aromatic oils. In a report made by the commissioner of patents. It was set forth that: "For many years it had been known that the vapor of sulfuric ether, when freely inhaled, would intoxicate as does alcohol when taken into the stomach, but that the former was much more temporary in its effects. But notwithstanding the records of its effects to this extent, which were familiar to so many, no surgeon had ever attempted to substitute it for the palliatives in common use previous to surgical operations. That, in view of these and other considerations, a patent had been granted for the discovery."

In 1846 an English patent was obtained. Morton soon began the attempt to sell office rights, as do the dentists of today, while the medical profession was then, as ever, antagonistic to patents, holding them to be subversive of general good. His patent was soon opposed and then generally infringed upon. Litigation followed without end, and the government stultified itself by refusing to recognize the validity of the patent issued by itself. And so, without any compensation to the discoverer, ether soon came into general use in this country as abroad. While receiving many congratulations from friends and humanitarians, Morton's success aroused the jealousy of some of his professional brethren, among them one Dr. Flagg, who commenced a terrible onslaught upon the new application of ether and its promoter. By his machinations a meeting of Boston dentists was called and a committee of twelve appointed to make a formal protest against anesthesia. This committee published a manifesto in the Boston Daily Advertiser, in which all sorts of untoward effects and unpleasant results were attributed to the new anesthetic.

This proclamation was spread broadcast, and did Morton, for the time, very much harm. Equally obstreperous was

Dr. Westcott, connected with the Dental College in Baltimore. He made fun of Morton's "sucking bottles," as his inhalers were dubbed; and in various of the medical and secular journals of the day, bitter, often foolish and absurd, attacks were made. The editors of the New Orleans Medical and Surgical Journal said:

"That the leading surgeons of Boston could be captivated by such an invention as this, heralded to the world under such auspices and upon such evidences of utility and safety as are presented by Dr. Bigelow, excites our amazement. Why, mesmerism, which is repudiated by the savants of Boston, has done a thousand times greater wonders, and without any of the dangers here threatened. What shall we see next?"

These and similar statements created a very strong prejudice against Morton, who, in December, 1846, sent to Washington, to a nephew of Dr. Warren, to endeavor to urge upon the government the advantages of employing ether in the army during the Mexican war, then in progress. The chief of the Bureau of Medicine and Surgery reported that the article might be of some service for use in large hospitals, but did not think it expedient for the department to incur any expense by introducing it into the general service; while the acting surgeon-general believed that the highly volatile character of the substance itself made it ill-adapted to the rough usage it would necessarily encounter upon the field of battle, and accordingly declined to recommend its use. In January of 1853, Morton demonstrated at the infirmary in Washington, before a congressional committee and others, the anesthetic effect of ether, which he continued through a dangerous and protracted surgical operation. This was the result of a challenge to compare the effects of nitrous oxide and those of ether, the advocates of the former not putting in an appearance.

The balance of Morton's life seems to have been spent in continued jangles. The government, having repudiated its own patent, was repeatedly besought by memorials and through the influence of members of Congress to bestow some testimonial upon or make some money return to Morton for his discovery. Several times he came near a realization of his hopes in this respect, when the action of some of his enemies or the termination of a congressional session, or some other accident, would doom him again to disappointment. The pages of evidence that were printed, the various reports issued through or by government officers, the memorials addressed from various individuals and societies, if all printed together, would make a large volume; but all of these were of no avail. Morton spent all his means, as he spent his energies and time, in futile endeavor to get pecuniary recognition of his discovery, but was doomed to disappointment. He seemed alike a victim of unfortunate circumstances and of treachery and animosity upon the part of his opponents. Especially did the fight wage warm between him and his friends and Jackson. Plots to ruin his business were repeatedly hatched and his life was made miserable in many ways. Mere temporary sops to wounded vanity and impaired fortune were the honorary degrees and the testimonials that came to him from various institutions of learning and foreign societies.

In 1850 both Morton and Jackson received from the French Academy prizes valued at 2,500 francs each. Finally, Morton fell into a state of nervous prostration, suffered from anxiety and insomnia, and in a fit of temporary aberration exposed himself in Central Park, New York, became unconscious, and was taken to St. Luke's hospital, dying just as he reached the institution, on the 15th of July, 1868. In Mount Auburn cemetery, in Boston, there stands a beautiful monument to William T. G. Morton, bearing this inscription: "Inventor and revealer of anesthetic inhalation, before whom in all time surgery was agony; by whom pain in surgery was averted and annulled; since whom science has control of pain."

Again, in the public garden in Boston there was erected, in 1867, a beautiful monument to the honor of the discoverer of ether, upon whom at that time they could not decide. Upon the front are these words: "To commemorate that the inhaling of ether causes insensibility to pain, first proven to the world at the Massachusetts General hospital, in Boston, October, A. D. 1846." Upon the right side are the words: "'Neither shall there be any more pain.'- Revelations." Upon the left: "'This also cometh forth from the Lord of Hosts, which is wonderful in counsel and excellent in working.'- Isaiah." And upon the other: "In gratitude for the relief of human suffering by the inhaling of ether, a citizen of Boston has erected this monument, A. D. 1867. The gift of Thomas Lee."

Summing up, then, the claims of our four contestants in the light of a collected history of the merits of each, it would appear that Wells first made public use of nitrous oxide gas for limited purposes, but failed to introduce it into general professional use. That Long, in an isolated rural practice, a few times used ether, with which he produced probably only partial insensibility to pain, and that he had apparently discontinued its use before learning of Morton's researches. That Jackson made no claim to the use of the agent on his own part, but simply of having suggested it to Morton. And, finally, that Morton quickly accepted the suggestion, made careful and scientific use thereof, but especially, and above all other things, first demonstrated to the world at large the capability and the safety of this agent as an absolute, reliable and efficient anesthetic. So, though Morton permitted his cupidity to run away with finer ethical considerations, and attached a higher pecuniary than humanitarian value to sulfuric ether, he, nevertheless, must be generally credited with having, to use the modern expression, "promoted" its introduction, and having shown to the world at large what an inestimably valuable therapeutic agent had been added to our resources for the control of pain.

The synthetic compound known as chloroform was discovered independently by three different observers between 1830 and 1832. These were respectively Guthrie, of Sackett's Harbor, N. Y.; Soubeiran, of France, and Liebig, of Germany.

The honor of introducing it to the profession as an anesthetic for surgical purposes is universally accorded to James Y. Simpson, then of Edinburgh. Yet claim was at one time advanced in favor of Surgeon-Major Furnell, of the Madras Army Medical Corps, who in the summer preceding the announcement of Simpson's brilliant discovery experimented with what is known as chloric ether, which is not an ether at all, but a solution of chloroform in alcohol. It is said that he found that it would produce the same results as sulfuric ether, with less unpleasant sensations, and suggested its use to Coote, a well-known London surgeon. However, such claims as those made in favor of Furnell are no more entitled to recognition than are those of Wells or Long in the matter of the introduction of ether to the public; for although individual observations were favorable to the compound, it never came to public notice on this surmise.

Sir James Y. Simpson was born in 1811, took the degree of doctor of medicine in 1832 and advanced rapidly in his professional career until, in January, 1847, he was appointed one of her majesty's physicians in Scotland. Having already obtained a large reputation, particularly in midwifery and gynecology, he directed his special attention toward the use of anesthetics in childbirth, and he had quickly recognized the value of sulfuric ether when introduced the previous year. He sought, however, for a substitute of equal power, having less disagreeable odor and unpleasant after effect. Upon inquiry of his friend Waldie, Master of Apothecaries Hall of Liverpool, if he knew of a substance likely to be of service in this direction, Waldie, familiar with the composition of chloric ether, suggested its active principle chloroform; with which Simpson experimented, and, upon the 4th of November, 1847, established its anesthetic properties. These he first made known to the Medico-Chirurgical Society of Edinburgh in a paper read November 10th. Three days later a public test was to have been made at the Royal Infirmary, but Simpson, who was to administer the chloroform, being unavoidably detained, the operation was done as heretofore without an anesthetic, and this patient died during the operation.

You can readily see that had this occurred under chloroform it would have been ascribed to the new drug, which would then and there have received its death blow. As it was, the first public trial took place two days later and the test was most successful.

One would think that such a boon as Simpson had here offered to the world would have been gratefully- not to say greedily- accepted by all. Simpson's position was such as to give the new anesthetic every advantage that his already great reputation could attach to it, and it became at once the agent in common use in midwifery practice. But the Scotch clergy of his day still possessed altogether too much of the old fanatic spirit of the church of the middle ages. One is never allowed to forget, in scanning the history of medicine, how bitterly the church has opposed, until recently, every advance in our science and our art. It was in A. D 995, for instance, that the son of one of the Venetian Doges was married, in Venice, to a sister of the emperor of the Eastern Roman Empire. At the marriage feast the princess produced a silver fork and gold spoon, table novelties which excited both amusing and angry comment. But the Venetian aristocracy took up with this new table fad, and forks and spoons as substitutes for fingers soon became the fashion. But the puissant church disapproved most strongly even of this arrangement, for priests went so far as to say, "to use forks was to deliberately insult the kind Providence which had given to man fingers on each hand." It was this same spirit that led the Scotch clergy to attack Simpson most vehemently and denounce him from their pulpits as one who violated the moral law, for they said: "Is it not ordained in Scripture, 'in sorrow shalt thou bring forth children?' and yet this man would introduce a substance calculated to mitigate this sorrow."

We of today can scarcely imagine the rancor with which these attacks were made for many months. Finally, however, these fanatic defenders of the faith were routed by a quotation from the same Scriptures in which they claimed to find their authority; for Simpson, most adroitly turning upon them with their own weapons, called their attention to the first chapter of Genesis, in which an account of Eve's creation appears, and reminded them that when Eve was formed from the rib of Adam, the Lord "caused a deep sleep to fall upon" him. So weak was their cause that with this single quotation their opposition subsided and within a week or two the entire Scotch clergy was silenced. Sir James Simpson received from his own government that which was never accorded to Morton: that is, due recognition of the great service he had rendered humanity. He died in 1870, and upon his bust, which stands in Westminster Abbey, are the following words: "To whose genius and beneficence the world owes the blessings derived from the use of chloroform for the relief of suffering."

It is scarcely necessary that I delay you now with an account of all of the other ethereal anesthetic agents which have from time to time been advocated since the memorable days to which I have devoted most of my time tonight. Two only are at present ever thought of- namely, bichlorid of methylene and bromide of ethyl- and these are used by only a few, though each has its advantages. It is well known that nearly all of the ethers have more or less of anesthetic property, coupled with many dangers and disadvantages. Sulfuric ether and chloroform hold the boards today as against any and all of their competitors. Nitrous oxide gas, as already mentioned, was known to and used by Wells, in Hartford. With the advent of ether this gas fell at once into disuse, to be revived some fifteen years after the death of Wells, mainly through the use of Dr. G. Q. Colton. Since this time its use has been quite universal, although confined for the main part to the offices of dentists.

Its great advantages are ease of administration and rapidity of recovery, making it especially useful for their purposes, while the difficulties attendant upon prolonged anesthesia by it makes it less useful for the surgeon. I will spend no further time upon it nor upon the subject save to do justice to modern anesthesia by a very different method and by means of a very different drug, which is today in so common use that we almost forget to mention the man to whom we owe it. I allude to Cocaine and its discoverer. Roller. Cocaine is now such a universally recognized local anesthetic that there is the best of reason for referring to it here- the more so because it affords another opportunity to do honor to a discoverer, who has rendered a most important service to not only our profession, but to the world in general.

This principal active constituent of cocoa leaves was discovered about 1860 by Niemann, and called by him cocaine. It is an alkaloid which combines with various acids in the formation of salts. It has the quality of benumbing raw and mucous surfaces, for which purpose it was applied first in 1862 by Schroff, and in 1868 by Moreno. In 1880, Van Aurap hinted that this property might some day be utilized. Karl Koller logically concluded from what was known about it that this anesthetic property could be taken advantage of for work about the eye, and made a series of experiments upon the lower animals, by which he established its efficiency and made a brilliant discovery. He reported his experiments to the Congress of German Oculists, at Heidelberg, In 1884. News of this was transmitted with great rapidity, and within a few weeks the substance was used all over the world. Its use spread rapidly to other branches of surgery, and cocaine local anesthesia became quickly an accomplished fact. More time was required to point out its disagreeable possibilities, its toxic properties and the like, but it now has an assured and most important place among anesthetic agents, and has been of the greatest use to probably 10 percent, of the civilized world. To Koller is entirely due the credit of establishing Its remarkable properties.

THE END